Indications for Diagnostic Procedures

TOPICS IN CLINICAL CARDIOLOGY

Series Editor: J. WILLIS HURST, M.D.

New Types of Cardiovascular Diseases
J. Willis Hurst, M.D.

Complications of Interventional Procedures
Jerre F. Lutz, M.D.

Indications for Diagnostic Procedures
Albert E. Raizner, M.D.

Cardiovascular Involvement in Systemic Diseases
J. David Talley, M.D.

Indications for Diagnostic Procedures

Albert E. Raizner, M.D.

Professor of Medicine
Baylor College of Medicine
Director, Cardiac Catheterization Laboratories
The Methodist Hospital
Houston, Texas

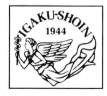

IGAKU-SHOIN New York • Tokyo

Published and distributed by

IGAKU-SHOIN Medical Publishers, Inc.
One Madison Avenue, New York, New York 10010

IGAKU-SHOIN Ltd.,
5-24-3 Hongo, Bunkyo-ku, Tokyo 113-91

Library of Congress Cataloging-in-Publication Data

Raizner, Albert E.
    Topics in clinical cardiology: indications for
diagnostic procedures / Albert E. Raizner.
       p.   cm.—(Topics in clinical cardiology)
    Includes bibliographical references and index.
    1. Heart—Diseases—Diagnosis.   2. Heart—Imaging. I. Title.
II. Series.
    [DNLM: 1. Cardiovascular Diseases—diagnosis. 2. Diagnostic
Imaging—methods. WG 141 R161t 1997]
    RC683.R24   1997
    616.1'20754—dc20
    DNLM/DLC
    for Library of Congress   96-30883
                                              CIP

ISBN: 0-89460-318-1   (New York)
ISBN: 4-260-14318-2   (Tokyo)

Printed and bound in the U.S.A.
10 9 8 7 6 5 4 3 2 1

Preface

During the past twenty-five years, the medical community has witnessed a technologic explosion affecting all aspects of medicine. No medical discipline, however, has benefited as much as cardiology and the cardiovascular sciences. Unparalleled in medical history is the capability of the modern physician to evaluate and diagnose the patient with suspected or known cardiovascular disease.

While the availability of tests and procedures which provide the keys to unlock the heretofore hidden secrets of the heart has imbued the modern cardiovascular physician with the power to find, to fix, and to follow cardiovascular disorders, it has also created an unprecedented level of responsibility of many physician groups to know and understand these tools, what to use, when to use them, and how to best utilize the information which they provide.

Though the cardiologist is most likely to deal with these tests and procedures on a daily basis, it behooves other physician groups to have comparable understanding of their indications and uses. For example, the cardiovascular surgeon and anesthesiologist must now become proficient in transesophageal echocardiography which has become an integral part of complex cardiovascular surgery; the internist must now know how to objectively assess for diastolic dysfunction, a heretofore elusive but nonetheless common disorder presenting with common symptoms.

But perhaps the greatest responsibility to learn and understand the cardiovascular diagnostic procedures befalls the primary care physician, the so-called "gatekeepers" in the new managed care environment, who must now develop a level of sophistication and knowledge comparable to the cardiovascular specialist with the diagnostic armamentarium available to maintain the high quality of care that the cardiac or potential cardiac patient has a right to expect.

Each chapter in this book focuses on a test or group of tests. Some, such as the chapters on Echocardiography (Dr. Quiñones), Nuclear Cardiology Testing (Dr. Verani), Coronary Angiography (Drs. Kleiman and Raizner) and Non-Cardiac Angiography (Dr. Raizner) represent frequently used procedures which have become highly refined and yet are ever expanding. Others, such as Positron Emission Tomography (Dr. McGhie) and Magnetic Resonance Imaging (Drs. Rokey and Vick) have important application but perhaps are not as well understood by the practicing community. Still others, such as the chapters on Transesophageal Echocardiography (Dr. Zoghbi) and Electrophysiologic Studies (Drs. Gallinghouse and Scheinman) are procedures whose growth and applicability show no signs of slowing. Finally, some such as the section on ultrafast CT in the chapter on Computed Tomography (Drs. Hedrick and Mahmarian) and the chapter on Coronary Doppler Flow Measurements (Dr. Kern) are in their infancy or early adolescence stage and still incompletely understood but are poised to take their places in the cardiovascular arena as important diagnostic tools.

Indications for Cardiovascular Diagnostic Procedures provides a concise update on these important "tools" and we hope will serve as an important adjunct to the many physicians whose professional responsibility requires an understanding of their use.

Albert E. Raizner, M.D.

DEDICATION

To my family: my wife, Andi; our parents,
Claire Raizner, Dave and Bea Boslow; our
children, Mike, Jeff, Susie, Mitchell . . .
and my new granddaughter, Kayla.

Acknowledgments

This book is one of a series of "Topics in Clinical Cardiology" edited by Dr. J. Willis Hurst. This series is one of many publications, monographs, and textbooks written or edited by Dr. J. Willis Hurst. These publications are one aspect of a career dedicated to the education and teaching of clinical medicine to students, residents, fellows, and colleagues by Dr. J. Willis Hurst. And this author (AER) is one of many thousands who has learned the science and art of being a doctor from Dr. J. Willis Hurst. His influence on the careers of so many physicians and on the practice of medicine and cardiology in general is gratefully acknowledged.

This editor also wishes to thank, with sincere appreciation, the chapter authors for their superb contributions to this edition.

Contributors

G. Joseph Gallinghouse, M.D.
Department of Medicine and the
   Cardiovascular Research Institute
University of California, San Francisco
San Francisco, California

Thomas D. Hedrick, M.D.
Clinical Assistant Professor
Department of Radiology
Baylor College of Medicine
Medical Director
Body MRI
The Methodist Hospital
Houston, Texas

Morton J. Kern, M.D.
Professor of Internal Medicine
Division of Cardiology
Director
J. G. Mudd Cardiac Catheterization Laboratory
St. Louis University Medical Center
St. Louis, Missouri

Neal S. Kleiman, M.D.
Associate Professor of Medicine
Baylor College of Medicine
Assistant Director, Cardiac Catheterization Laboratories
The Methodist Hospital
Houston, Texas

John J. Mahmarian, M.D.
Associate Professor of Medicine
Baylor College of Medicine
Assistant Director
Nuclear Cardiology Laboratory
The Methodist Hospital
Houston, Texas

A. Iain McGhie, M.D.
Assistant Professor of Medicine
Director of Nuclear Cardiology
University of Texas and Hermann Hospital
Houston, Texas

Miguel A. Quiñones, M.D.
Professor of Medicine
Baylor College of Medicine
Director, Echocardiography Laboratory
The Methodist Hospital
Houston, Texas

Albert E. Raizner, M.D.
Professor of Medicine
Baylor College of Medicine
Director, Cardiac Catheterization Laboratories
The Methodist Hospital
Houston, Texas

Roxann Rokey, M.D.
Clinical Associate Professor of Medicine
University of Wisconsin
Department of Cardiology
Marshfield Clinic
Marshfield, Wisconsin

Melvin M. Scheinman, M.D.
Department of Medicine and the
   Cardiovascular Research Institute
University of California, San Francisco
San Francisco, California

Mario S. Verani, M.D.
Professor of Medicine
Baylor College of Medicine
Director, Nuclear Cardiology
The Methodist Hospital
Houston, Texas

G. Wesley Vick, M.D.
Assistant Professor of Pediatrics
Division of Pediatric Cardiology
Baylor College of Medicine
Houston, Texas

William A. Zoghbi, M.D.
Associate Professor of Medicine
   Section of Cardiology
Director, Echocardiography Research
Baylor College of Medicine
Houston, Texas

Contents

— Section 1 —
NONINVASIVE DIAGNOSTIC PROCEDURES

—1—

Indications for Echocardiography

Miguel A. Quiñones M.D.

DESCRIPTION OF TECHNIQUE

Echocardiography, also known as cardiac ultrasound, is a noninvasive diagnostic technique that uses reflected ultrasound waves to image the heart in motion. Repeated pulses of sound waves in the 2 to 7 MHz range are used to create a sound beam which is then stirred across a 45 to 100° arc to generate an image. The principle behind ultrasound imaging is that the speed of sound in tissue is constant and therefore, the time required for a reflected sound wave (or echo) to return to the transducer is proportional to the distance from transducer to reflecting tissue. Because the sound waves are scanned through a two-dimensional plane, the images obtained are tomographic, i.e., they provide a cross-sectional anatomy of the heart and great vessels. Multiple two-dimensional tomographic planes are produced by directing the sound waves from several positions (or examining windows) within the chest, subcostal region, suprasternal notch or esophagus, and from these positions, orienting the transducer into the desired view.

The following are the diagnostic techniques currently available within the field of echocardiography:

Two-Dimensional and M-Mode Echocardiography (2D)

Two-dimensional images are produced by the summation of ultrasound scan lines that are swiped form left to right and blended together by an image processing algorithm. The echoes returning from a selected scan line can be recorded in motion in

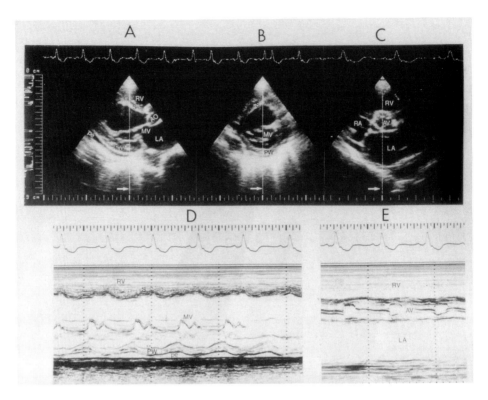

Figure 1.1. Two-dimensional (2D) views of the heart. (A) Parasternal long axis view. (B) Parasternal short axis view of the left ventricle (LV). (C) Short axis view of the aortic root (AO) and left atrium (LA). Panels (D) and (E) illustrate the M-mode recordings derived from the cursor lines shown in A and B, respectively. Note the small posterior pericardial effusion (pe) in A and D. Other abbreviations: RV = right ventricle; MV = mitral valve; S = septum; PW = posterior wall; AV = aortic valve.

what is known as an M-mode. Because of its superior time resolution, M-mode is used to plot the motion of structures within the heart such as a cardiac valve (Figure 1.1). Two-dimensional echo is the main stem of echocardiography. It provides tomographic images of the heart chambers, including the left ventricle (LV), the valves, and the great vessels.

Doppler Echocardiography

This technology makes use of the Doppler principle to evaluate blood flow velocity (V) within the heart and great vessels. The Doppler principle states that the frequency of reflected ultrasound is shifted by a moving target such as red blood cells. The magnitude of this Doppler shift relates to the velocity of the blood cells while the polarity of the shift reflects the direction of blood flow toward (positive) or away (negative) from the transducer. Currently, Doppler echocardiography consists of two modalities: spectral Doppler which consists of pulsed (PW) and continuous wave

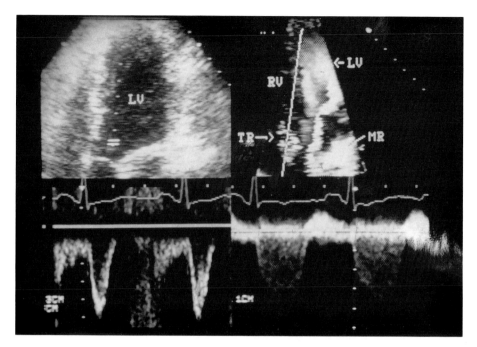

Figure 1.2.   Left upper quadrant shows a 2D echo image of the LV in the apical long axis view with a pulsed Doppler sample volume (*parallel lines*) positioned in the LV outflow tract. The quadrant below illustrates the pulsed Doppler spectral tracing of the LV outflow velocity. On the right upper quadrant, color Doppler obtained from the apical four-chamber view shows a small jet of tricuspid regurgitation (TR) and a jet of mitral regurgitation (MR) that covers most of the area of the left atrium. A cursor line is seen directed at the TR jet from which a continuous wave spectral Doppler tracing is derived and shown on the right lower quadrant. The peak velocity of this TR jet is 3.5 m/sec (velocity scale is set at 1 m/sec). Using the modified Bernoulli equation results in an estimated pressure difference between right ventricle (RV) and right atrium of 49 mm Hg.

(CW) Doppler, and color flow Doppler (Figure 1.2). Pulsed Doppler records the blood flow velocity within discrete areas inside the heart or in a blood vessel but is limited by the aliasing phenomenon that prevents it from measuring velocities beyond a given threshold (or Nyquist limit). Continuous wave Doppler uses continuous, rather than pulsatile sound waves, and is not affected by aliasing. Consequently, CW Doppler is capable of recording very high flow velocities but is unable to localize the site of origin of these velocities within the pathway of the sound beam. Color flow Doppler makes use of the pulsed Doppler technology but with the addition of multiple gates or regions of interest within the path of the sound beam. In each of these regions, an estimate of the flow velocity is made and superimposed on the two-dimensional image in the form of shades of red or blue colors depending on the direction of flow toward or away from the transducer, respectively. All three Doppler modalities are incorporated within the ultrasound system and are used in conjunction with 2D imaging.

The clinical utility of Doppler echocardiography is divided in two categories, detection of valvular lesions and intracardiac shunts, and quantification of flow velocities. For detection purposes, all three modalities perform well with high sensitivity and specificity. However, color flow Doppler is the preferred technique for regurgitant valve lesions and intracardiac shunts because it provides a spatial display of the abnormal flow in the two-dimensional plane. Measurements of flow velocity are primarily obtained with PW or CW Doppler. PW Doppler is used primarily to measure velocities of laminar flows across normal valves or vessels in order to assess cardiac function or calculate flow. Continuous wave Doppler, on the other hand, is used to measure high velocities across small areas such as stenotic or regurgitant valve orifices. These velocities are converted into pressure gradients by applying the simplified Bernoulli equation, pressure gradient $= 4V^2$.

Stress Echocardiography

Stress echocardiography applies 2D echo to visualize the LV and detect regional wall motion abnormalities during interventions known to cause ischemia. The test is used to detect coronary artery disease (CAD) or evaluate patients with known CAD for the presence of ischemia.

Transesophageal Echocardiography (TEE)

This newer technology uses an ultrasound transducer mounted at the tip of an endoscope that is passed into the esophagus and stomach to visualize the heart and great vessels. Because of the proximity of the esophagus to the heart, a higher frequency transducer can be used resulting in images of higher resolution. The transducer is capable of providing 2D and M-mode, PW, CW, and color flow Doppler. TEE is used in patients with suboptimal quality of images from the standard transthoracic approach or to visualize better structures that are posteriorly located and in close proximity to the esophagus.

DEVELOPMENTAL PERSPECTIVES

Diagnostic ultrasound was introduced in 1955 by Edler[1] but it was not until the mid to late 1960s that the technology improved sufficiently to be of clinical utility. A piezoelectric crystal vibrates and emits sound waves when electrically stimulated, and produces an electrical current when mechanically stretched by the reflected sound waves. The first instruments operated using a single ultrasound piezoelectric crystal that alternated between producing and receiving sound waves and could be used to generate an M-mode recording of intracardiac structures. The transducer was positioned along the left sternal border and directed blindly into the heart to obtain the desired recording. The reflected structures appeared as moving waves that made sense only to the trained echocardiographer. During the decade of the 1970s, a body of knowledge was accumulated that allowed the application of M-mode echocardiography to the noninvasive evaluation of valvular abnormalities, detection of pericardial effusion, and assessment of cardiac chamber size and LV function, all of which were limited by the "ice pick" view provided by the technique.

In the mid 1970s two-dimensional echocardiography was introduced. The first systems created a 2D image by mechanically oscillating (or rotating) the sound waves produced by a single crystal transducer. Initially the images were limited to 45° arc but these were rapidly expanded to 90° or more. In the first systems, the multiple scan lines that produced the image were visible but by the late 1970s, digital scan converters were introduced that blended the scan lines with each other and produced a better quality image that was pleasant to the eye and could be frozen in the screen and printed. Around the same time, the phase array technology was introduced. This technology consists of a transducer containing many small piezoelectric crystals that are triggered electronically in sequence so as to stir the scan lines across a 90° arc. To this day, both technologies, mechanical and phase-array, have continued to evolve improving both penetration and image quality. Phase-array systems are more complex and expensive but provide a higher resolution image. The mechanical systems have improved with the development of the annular array technology by which ultrasound crystals are mounted in concentric rings that are electronically triggered to produce a sound beam that is then mechanically oscillated. Developments in the processing of the returning echoes led to the addition of spectral Doppler and later, color Doppler.

TECHNICAL CONSIDERATIONS

Ultrasound equipment is small and portable enough to allow the procedure to be performed in a laboratory or at the bedside. Both 2D and Doppler recordings are obtained with the same transducer and from similar windows of examination. Echocardiography is usually performed by a specialized technician or sonographer with the exception of TEE which is performed by a physician–echocardiographer. Although it is not common for the physician to routinely perform echocardiographic studies, he/she must be available to supervise the sonographer and perform the procedure if required, particularly in patients with complex pathology.

For routine transthoracic studies, the only personnel required is the sonographer and the physician–echocardiographer who interprets the test. In the case of TEE, the physician is frequently accompanied by a sonographer and a nurse who cares for the patient during the procedure. Likewise, stress echocardiography requires the presence of a sonographer to obtain the echo images, a technician or nurse to monitor the electrocardiogram, and a physician to supervise the procedure. A nurse should be available to administer drugs or a particular pharmacologic agent used as stressor. Furthermore, the laboratory should be fully equipped to handle cardiac emergencies including an arrest.

Echocardiography is limited primarily by the quality of the images obtained and the expertise of the echocardiographer interpreting the procedure. Image quality is dependent on transducer frequency, technical qualities of the transducer and ultrasound system, the level of ultrasound penetration required to reach the cardiac structures, the ultrasound density of structures proximal to the target structure, and the expertise of the sonographer. The axial resolution of the image (i.e., the capacity to distinguish two targets that are very close to each other) relates directly to the emitted frequency of sound. Unfortunately, higher frequency sound waves penetrate less into tissue than lower frequency waves. Thus, when studying adult patients a trade-off is often made between image resolution and penetration. This is particularly true for cardiac structures at the far end of the ultrasound field such as the left atrium or descending thoracic aorta. These structures are better visualized from the esophagus using TEE.

Whenever ultrasound passes through a dense structure, the sound waves are attenuated so that less of them are available distal to the structure. In addition, reverberation of ultrasound waves within a dense structure produces artifacts of echoes that are interpreted by the machine as originating distal to the structure. An example of this phenomenon is when a mechanical prosthesis precludes adequate visualization of the left atrium. One particular source of attenuation is air. The presence of air around or proximal to the heart severely limits the resolution of the image.

The speed of sound within the body is constant. Therefore, time is spent in awaiting for the sound to reflect and come back. Additional time is needed for processing the echoes and to derive the images and the Doppler information. The end result is that there are limits to how fast an image can be created, which in turn affects the frame rate (or temporal resolution) of the system. The more complex the processing portion is (for instance, color is more complex than 2D alone), the slower the frame rate. Likewise, the frame rate is limited by the width and the depth of the image plane. Despite these limitations, echocardiography still provides better time resolution than most other noninvasive imaging techniques.

INDICATIONS AND USES

This chapter will focus on the indications for transthoracic 2D, Doppler, and stress echocardiography. It is impossible within the limits of a chapter to discuss every possible application of echocardiography and thus, we will emphasize the primary ones and group them according to categories. These indications are well summarized in the American College of Cardiology/American Heart Association Task Force report on guidelines for the clinical application of echocardiography.[2] The indications for TEE are discussed in Chapter 6.

Evaluation of Cardiac Function

Evaluation of the Left Ventricle

Echocardiography is currently the noninvasive method most commonly used for the evaluation of left ventricular size, hypertrophy, and function. The clinical scenarios where 2D is often required to assess LV function are listed in Table 1.1. The left ventricle is visualized in multiple views, the most common ones being the parasternal long and short axis, and the apical four and two-chamber views (Figure 1.3). From these views one can appreciate the contraction of the different walls of the

TABLE 1.1. Indications for Echocardiography: Cardiac Function

Indications	*Common Clinical Scenarios*
1. Evaluation of LV function	
2D: LV size, hypertrophy, EF, regional wall motion abnormalities	Recent or old myocardial infarction
	Abnormal ECG such as left bundle branch block, LVH, pathologic Q waves, repolarization abnormalities, etc.
	Cardiomegaly by chest x-ray
	Systemic hypertension with suspicion of LVH
	Prior to major surgery in patients with suspected heart disease
	Screening for familial hypertrophic or dilated cardiomyopathy
Doppler: Cardiac output, PA pressure, diastolic function, estimates of LV filling pressures	Congestive heart failure
	Dyspnea
	Unexplained edema/ascites
	Critically ill patients with hypotension or shock
2. Evaluation of LA, RA, or RV	
2D: Chamber size, RV function inferior vena cava	Atrial fibrillation
	ECG evidence of RVH or conduction abnormalities
	Radiographic evidence of enlarged RV, RA, or pulmonary arteries
Doppler: PA pressures, estimates of RA pressures	Suspicion of pulmonary hypertension
	Unexplained right heart failure

LV = left ventricle; EF = ejection fraction; PA = pulmonary artery; LA = left auricle; RA = right auricle; RV = right ventricle; LVH = left ventricular hypertrophy; RVH = right ventricular hypertrophy.

ventricle. The size of the chamber can be assessed by measuring cavity dimensions or determining volumes. The latter is done by tracing the endocardial contour of the LV cavity in the apical views and applying formulas based on geometric models.[3] Measurements of LV volumes or cavity dimensions are important in the evaluation of patients with dilated cardiomyopathy, valvular regurgitation, and in those recovering from a myocardial infarction (MI), since excessive LV dilatation (or remodeling) has been associated with a worse prognosis.[4–7]

Left ventricular ejection fraction (EF), defined as stroke volume divided by end-diastolic volume, is the most frequently used parameter of LV systolic performance. Although EF can be visually estimated, the method requires a very high level of expertise by the echocardiographer. Quantitative techniques are currently available to calculate EF with results that correlate well with radionuclide and angiographic standards,[8–11] and should be preferred to the subjective estimation. It is worthwhile noting that all methods of measuring EF, whether invasive or noninvasive, have inherent sources of error and consequently a certain degree of variability. This was recently demonstrated by Naik et al. in a metanalysis of studies in the literature comparing echo and nuclear methods to each other and to angiography.[11]

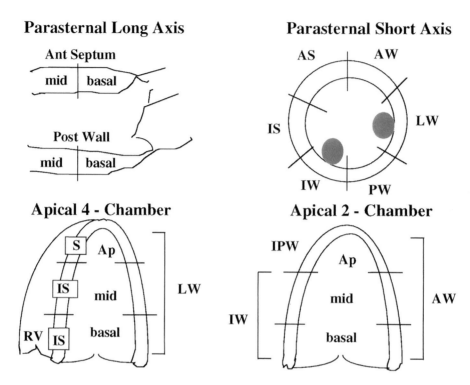

Figure 1.3. Diagrammatic illustration of the four views commonly used in the evaluation of the left ventricle. The parasternal long axis provides a view of the basal and middle (mid) segments of the anterior septum (AS) and posterior (post) wall. The parasternal short axis is obtained at the level of the papillary muscles and provides a cross-sectional view of all of the middle segments of the left ventricle. The apical four-chamber view visualizes the basal, middle, and apical segments of the lateral wall (LW) and septum (S; IS = inferior septum). The apical two-chamber view visualizes the basal, middle, and apical segments of the anterior wall (AW) and inferior wall (IW); IPW = inferoposterior.

    Evaluation of regional wall motion is important in patients with ischemic heart disease. Wall motion is assessed subjectively using both the extent of endocardial motion and systolic wall thickening. Segmental division of the left ventricle is most commonly performed following the recommendations of the American Society of Echocardiography (Figure 1.3).[3] The walls of the ventricle and the septum are divided into basilar, mid, and apical segments and each segment classified as: 1 = normal, 2 = hypokinetic, 3 = akinetic, or 4 = dyskinetic. A wall motion score index is derived as the sum of the segmental scores divided by the number of segments visualized.[3] To date, no quantitative technique has been capable of surpassing the accuracy of a wall motion score when properly performed. Segmental wall motion scores have been used to quantitate the extent of ischemia during stress echocardiography, and the magnitude of improvement in regional wall motion following thrombolytic therapy or coronary angioplasty in patients with acute myocardial infarction.[12–14] In acute MI, the wall motion score is an index of severity of LV dysfunction that predicts in-hospital and one-year mortality.[15–17]

Echocardiography is the noninvasive method most commonly used to assess left ventricular hypertrophy (LVH) and in particular, establish the diagnosis of hypertrophic cardiomyopathy. The severity of LVH has been recently shown to be an independent predictor of poor clinical outcome, including death, in asymptomatic populations[18] and in patients with hypertension or coronary artery disease.[19–22] The best echocardiographic index of LV hypertrophy is LV mass which is calculated from cavity dimensions and wall thickness measurements. Several studies have clearly demonstrated the superiority of echocardiography over electrocardiography (ECG) in the detection of LV hypertrophy.[23–24]

Evaluation of Other Heart Chambers

The size of the left and right atria can be accurately evaluated by echocardiography using measured dimensions of the chambers or volume estimates. On the other hand, the right ventricle has a complicated geometry and consequently, derivation of volumes is fraught with inaccuracies. The size of this chamber is usually evaluated by the internal dimensions of the cavity.[25] Consequently, there are no current good methods of determining right ventricular (RV) ejection fraction. Nevertheless, one can evaluate subjectively the wall motion of the RV free wall and grade ventricular function as normal, mild, moderate, or severely depressed. Elevations of systolic or diastolic RV pressures induce alterations in the curvature of the interventricular septum, as seen in the short axis view which can be helpful in evaluating the severity of these hemodynamic abnormalities. Increasing systolic pressures flattens the curvature of the septum during systole, while increasing diastolic pressures (i.e., volume overload) flattens the septum during diastole. Clinical situations where echocardiography is commonly used to assess the atria or right ventricle are listed in Table 1.1.

Application of Doppler

Recordings of intracardiac flow velocities by Doppler add a hemodynamic complement to the evaluation provided by 2D echo. Stroke volume and cardiac output can be accurately derived as the product of the flow velocity across the aortic annulus and the cross-sectional area of the annulus (Figure 1.2).[26] The latter is calculated from the annulus diameter measured from the 2D image. Alternatively, stroke volume can also be determined at the mitral and/or pulmonic annulus. These other sites are useful in the presence of regurgitant valve lesions or intracardiac shunts (see below). In patients with hypertrophic cardiomyopathy, Doppler is utilized to detect intracavitary gradients and evaluate the severity of the outflow obstruction.[27]

Pulmonary artery (PA) systolic pressure is estimated from the peak velocity of tricuspid regurgitation (TR) is the absence of pulmonic valve stenosis (Figure 1.2).[28] The TR velocity is converted into the pressure difference between RV and RA using the modified Bernoulli equation, pressure gradient = $4V^2$, and the systolic RV (or PA) pressure is calculated by adding an estimate of RA pressure. The latter is derived by evaluating the degree of inspiratory collapse of the inferior vena cava[29] and/or the magnitude of antegrade flow velocity in the hepatic vein.[30] The frequent occurrence of mild TR in cardiac patients, and even in normal subjects, facilitates the wide application of this method. Whenever TR is not well recorded by Doppler, the

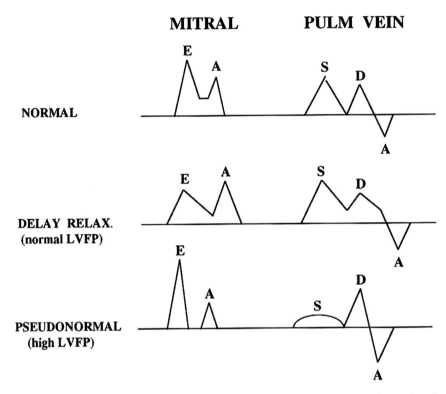

Figure 1.4. Diagrammatic illustration of the three common patterns of mitral and pulmonary (pulm) vein velocities that relate to diastolic function. Relax = relaxation; LVFP = left ventricular filling pressures. See text for definitions.

strength of the signal can be enhanced by injecting agitated saline intravenously. The microbubbles in the solution increase the ultrasound backscatter intensifying the amplitude of the TR signal.[31]

Flow velocity across the mitral valve and in the pulmonary veins provides significant insight into the diastolic function of the left ventricle (Figure 1.4). The two common diastolic abnormalities observed in cardiac patients are impairment of LV relaxation with normal filling pressures and impaired relaxation with increased chamber stiffness and high filling pressures. In the former, the transmitral velocity has a pattern of reduced early flow velocity (E), prolonged isovolumic relaxation time (IVRT; time from end of aortic flow to onset of mitral) and deceleration time (time from the E-velocity to an extrapolation of the descending slope to the zero baseline), with an increase in the velocity during atrial (A) contraction. The end result is an E/A ratio <1.0.[32] The pulmonary vein velocity shows a pattern of greater antegrade systolic (S) than diastolic (D) flow velocity.[33] Impaired relaxation is seen with normal aging, ischemia, LV hypertrophy (other than athlete's), increased afterload, and with any form of myocardial disease.[34] As LV stiffness and filling pressures increase, so do the E-velocity and E/A ratio. IVRT and deceleration time shorten and the A-velocity tends to decrease. The pattern resembles that seen in normal young subjects and thus has been called "pseudonormal".[32,34,35] In contrast to the normal pattern, the "pseudonormal" pattern is seen in patients with clinical and echocardiographic evidence of heart disease such as LV hypertrophy, LA enlargement, abnormal EF and/or regional wall motion, who often have symptoms of heart failure. Furthermore, the pulmonary vein velocity in these patients changes to a pattern of reduced antegrade systolic flow with accentuation of the retrograde A-velocity during atrial contraction.[33,36,37]

The patterns just described are dynamic and patients move from one to the other in response to instantaneous changes in filling pressures. Consequently, one can use Doppler to estimate filling pressures in patients suspected of having heart failure and to follow the effect of therapy on the filling pressures.[35,38,39] The technique works well even in patients with normal systolic performance and heart failure due to diastolic dysfunction. Likewise, estimates of cardiac output and PA systolic pressure are exquisitely sensitive to changes induced by therapy. This is true even when the 2D echo fails to demonstrate changes in chamber size or ejection fraction. The clinical situations where Doppler is recommended as part of a cardiac evaluation study are listed in Table 1.1; as expected they are similar to conditions where an invasive hemodynamic study would be desirable.

Stress Echocardiography

The purpose of stress echo is the detection of regional and global left ventricular dysfunction during an intervention known to induce ischemia. This is based on the concept that reversible myocardial contractile dysfunction is a highly sensitive marker of ischemia that precedes both ECG changes and chest pain. The two common interventions used are exercise and intravenous infusion of a pharmacologic agent that induces ischemia in the presence of a significant coronary artery stenosis. From a technical standpoint, the application of stress echo has been enhanced by the availability of digital frame grabbers that capture one or more cardiac cycles from each of the views at rest and during stress, and play them back in a cine-loop format (Figure 1.5). The images can be viewed side-by-side on a split or quad screen, facilitating the detection of new wall motion abnormalities.

Exercise echocardiography is performed either on a treadmill or a supine or upright bicycle. When treadmill is used, 2D images are obtained at rest and immediately after exercise. An attractive feature of the post-treadmill exercise echo is that it is combined with the same treadmill test that has been extensively used in the evaluation of CAD patients. In addition to the echocardiographic data, one obtains important information concerning exercise tolerance and ECG changes. Performing the exercise echo on a bicycle has the advantage of allowing the 2D echo views to be obtained during and at peak exercise, thus theoretically enhancing the detection of ischemia, particularly in an area that might recover quickly after termination of exercise. No real advantage exist between upright and supine bicycle although we prefer the latter mostly because of the ease with which one can add Doppler if desired to assess flow velocity dynamics.

Pharmacologic agents are currently available that will stress the heart and induce ischemia in patients with significant CAD who are not candidates for exercise testing. These agents are divided into two categories. The first are catecholamine-like agents that induce a tachycardia with increased inotropic stimulation and thus induce ischemia by a mechanism analogous to exercise, i.e., an imbalance between myocardial oxygen demands and supply. The most frequently used agent

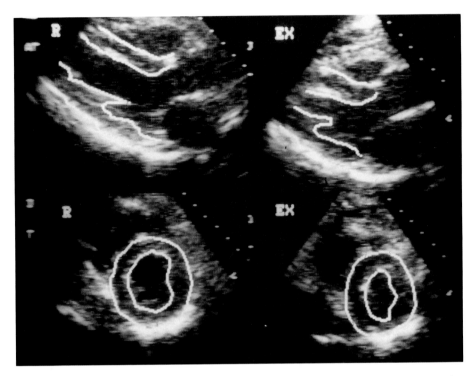

Figure 1.5.   Quad screen presentation of digitized images of the left ventricle on cine-loop during an exercise echocardiogram. The parasternal long-axis views are shown on top and the short-axis views below; rest (R) images are on the left and exercise (EX) images on the right. These images are normally played back through a computer for analysis of wall motion. The end-systolic frames are illustrated with the inner (or endocardial) and outer contours of the myocardium highlighted. Notice the reduction in end-systolic cavity size (or volume) with exercise and the increase in thickness of the walls.

in this category is dobutamine. The second category consists of coronary arteriolar vasodilators that normally increase myocardial blood flow by 3 to 5-fold. In the presence of critical coronary artery stenosis, these drugs produce a maldistribution of flow away from the affected area and into regions perfused by normal coronary arteries. Furthermore, within the affected region, flow is shifted toward the subepicardial area and away from the subendocardium, resulting in subendocardial ischemia.[40] The two drugs commonly used in this category are dipyridamole and adenosine.

By now there is extensive experience with stress echo.[41–50] The sensitivity of the test for detection of significant CAD ranges between 60% and 95% depending on: (1) choice of test (exercise and dobutamine are generally more sensitive than dipyridamole or adenosine), (2) heart rate achieved during exercise or dobutamine, (3) prevalence of single-vessel versus multi-vessel disease, (4) criteria used for defining significant coronary artery stenosis (i.e., ≥50% versus ≥70% diameter stenosis), and (5) criteria used for defining a positive test. The specificity ranges between 68% and 100% depending on the criteria used for defining a positive result. Failure to develop a hyperdynamic wall motion with exercise or dobutamine has been used by

TABLE 1.2. Indications for Stress Echocardiography

Indications	Common Clinical Scenarios	Preferred Mode of Stress
1. Detection of CAD (>50% stenosis)	Chest pain syndromes Positive exercise ECG done for screening purposes in asymptomatic patients with several risk factors	Exercise Pharmacologic if patient cannot exercise
2. Assess functional severity of CAD (Symptoms, onset of ischemia, extent of ischemia)	Chest pain syndromes Patient with known CAD	Exercise
3. Risk stratification (Presence and extent of ischemia, EF, LV volumes)	Patient with known CAD and minimal or no symptoms Following a noncomplicated myocardial infarction Patient with known or suspected CAD prior to major surgery	Exercise Pharmacologic if patient cannot exercise
4. Evaluate results of PTCA/CABG (Detection of ischemia)	Patients with prior PTCA or CABG with suspicion of recurrent ischemia	Exercise Pharmacologic if patient cannot exercise
5. Assessment of myocardial viability in patients with resting RWMA	Postmyocardial infarction Patient with chronic CAD and LV dysfunction	Dobutamine

CAD = coronary artery disease; EF = ejection fraction; LV = left ventgricular; PTCA = percutaneous transluminal coronary angioplasty; CABG = coronary artery bypass graft surgery; RWMA = regional wall motion abnormality.

some laboratories as an indicator of ischemia. Although sensitivity may be enhanced, the specificity of the test is lower when this criterion is used, particularly in elderly patients. In some patients with CAD, resting wall motion may be abnormal due to previous myocardial infarction or chronic ischemia–hibernation (see below). Using this finding increases the sensitivity for CAD detection but lowers the specificity since abnormal regional wall motion can be seen in patients with primary cardiomyopathy.

The indications for stress echocardiography are listed in Table 1.2 and are similar to those of stress perfusion imaging SPECT (single-photon emission computed tomography) thallium or sestamibi. The indications are divided into five categories: (1) detection of CAD, (2) evaluation of functional severity, (3) risk stratification, (4) evaluation of the effects of revascularization therapy, and (5) assessment of myocardial viability. In the first category, the most common use of stress echo is for detection of CAD in patients with chest pain syndromes in whom conventional treadmill ECG is known to be less accurate. These consist of women, patients with resting ECG abnormalities, and those suspected of having single-vessel CAD. Another common indication is when a positive treadmill ECG is suspected to be false-positive.

This occurs more commonly in asymptomatic men undergoing screening for CAD. The functional severity of CAD in a given patient can be assessed in terms of duration of exercise, presence of symptoms during the test, and extent of ischemia as determined by the wall motion abnormalities.

Stress echocardiography is uniquely suited for risk stratification since it can assess resting ejection fraction and detect ischemia in the same setting. The three groups of patients for whom risk stratification is important are those with chronic stable angina, patients surviving a noncomplicated MI, and those undergoing a major noncardiac surgical procedure. A growing body of literature is showing the value of exercise and pharmacologic stress echocardiography in discriminating between patients at low versus high risk of subsequent ischemic events and death.[51–55] Preliminary observations in our laboratory indicate that in ambulatory patients undergoing post-treadmill exercise echo, the combination of echocardiographic and ECG findings can be used to predict different event rates over a follow-up period of 5 yr.[56]

The most recent application of stress echo and in particular dobutamine echo, is for detection of viable myocardium in patients with resting left ventricular dysfunction.[57–59] When resting regional wall motion abnormalities are due to chronic ischemia and hibernation, they often recover following revascularization and thus, accurate detection of these regions has important clinical connotations. The rationale behind the use of doubutamine echo is that viable myocardium usually responds to dobutamine stimulation at lower doses of the agent. As the dose is increased beyond 20 μm/kg/min, the transient improvement in wall motion reverts to worsening as ischemia supervenes. This biphasic response has been recently demonstrated to be highly predictive of recovery of function following revascularization.[59]

In comparison with radionuclide perfusion imaging techniques, stress echo has the advantage of a lower cost, lack of radiation, and availability of additional information concerning LV size and function. The studies that have compared both techniques in the same patient have found comparable sensitivities for CAD detection when exercise or dobutamine is used.[43,44,60] In contrast, the sensitivity is superior for the perfusion studies when dipyridamole or adenosine is used. In general, specificity of stress echo has been slightly better than that of SPECT thallium or sestamibi. Preliminary data from our laboratory indicates that in an ambulatory patient population, exercise echo and SPECT thallium have similar accuracy in identifying patients at different risks of future ischemic events.[56] Studies are currently underway to assess the accuracy of stress echo versus myocardial perfusion imaging for the evaluation of myocardial viability.

Evaluation of Valvular Heart Disease

Echocardiography is currently the method of choice for the evaluation of patients with valvular heart disease. Valvular calcification and other structural abnormalities are readily apparent and the etiology of the valvular abnormality, whether congenital or acquired, is often recognized. In addition, echocardiography is used to assess the impact of the valvular lesion (or lesions) on the function of the left and right ventricle, and on left and right atrial size, all of which are important in making

TABLE 1.3. Indications for Echocardiography: Valvular, Endocarditis, and Intracardiac Masses

Indications	Common Clinical Scenarios
1. Evaluation of valvular lesions	

2D: Structural abnormalities, LV function, LA, RV and RA size
Doppler: Functional severity, PA pressures, estimates of RA pressures
	Heart murmur suggestive of valvular disease
	Known valvular heart disease
	  a. Evaluation of severity
	  b. Assessment of cardiac function
	Serial evaluation after valve repair or replacement
	Suspicion of prosthetic valve dysfunction

2. Endocarditis	
2D: Vegetations, abscesses, LV function (TEE is superior to transthoracic) Doppler: Assess regurgitant lesions, detect fistulae	Unexplained fever and heart murmur Septic emboli Bacteremia in a patient with valvular or congenital heart disease Patient with prosthetic valve and unexplained fever
3. Intracardiac masses	
2D: Detection, location, size, morphology, mobility Doppler: Impairment of valvular function, look for evidence of vascularity within the mass	Embolic episode Heart murmurs Dyspnea

therapeutic decisions. The common clinical situations where echocardiography is used to assess valvular function are listed in Table 1.3.

All of the Doppler modalities are applied when evaluating patients with valvular abnormalities. While regurgitant lesions are usually well detected with color flow Doppler, accurate assessment of their severity requires a careful integration of data derived from color Doppler, PW and CW Doppler. Color Doppler provides an appreciation for the area of regurgitant velocity within the receiving chamber in a given 2D plane (Figure 1.2).[61,62] This regurgitant jet area, however, is subject to multiple technical and physiologic sources of errors and should be used with caution.[62] On the other hand, a more accurate assessment of severity of regurgitation can be achieved by evaluating the size of the regurgitant jet velocity at or just distal to the valve orifice. In aortic and mitral regurgitation, the proximal width and cross-sectional area of the regurgitant jet relate well to the severity of the lesion.[63,64] In mitral regurgitation (MR), examination of the flow pattern proximal to the regurgitant valve can also provide quantitation of regurgitant severity. Proximal flow acceleration occurs with the isovelocity "surfaces" assuming a hemispherical or hemielliptical shape adjacent to the regurgitant orifice (Figure 1.6). The color flow image allows identification of the proximal isovelocity surface area at which the velocity is equal to the aliasing velocity. This velocity and the radius of the hemiellipse are used to derive the regurgitant flow and the effective regurgitant orifice area (Figure 1.6).[65] The latter is calculated as regurgitant flow divided by the velocity of regurgitation measured with CW Doppler. One can also calculate regurgitant volume using PW

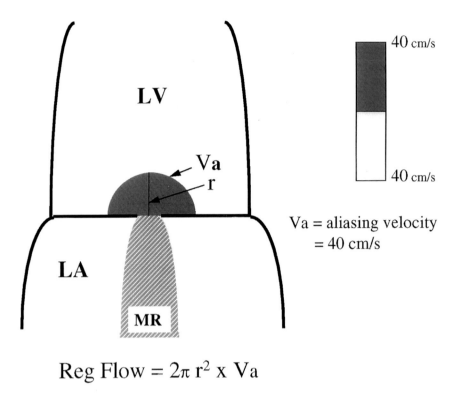

$$\text{Reg Flow} = 2\pi \; r^2 \; x \; Va$$

Figure 1.6. Diagrammatic illustration of the area of proximal acceleration as seen by color Doppler in a patient with significant mitral regurgitation (MR). Red colors are illustrated as dark gray and blue colors as light gray while the mosaic color appearance of the MR jet is illustrated as diagonal shades of gray. In this example the aliasing (or Nyquist) velocity is 40 cm/sec. The proximal isovelocity surface of acceleration, demarcated by the aliasing velocity, is hemispheric in geometry and thus its area can be derived as $2\pi \; r^2$. Consequently, the regurgitant (Reg) flow can be determined as this area multiplied by the aliasing velocity.

Doppler as stroke volume across the regurgitant valve minus stroke volume measured at a distant site. Regurgitant fraction is calculated as regurgitant volume divided by the volume across the regurgitant valve.[66] In aortic regurgitation, the regurgitant jet velocity by CW reflects the instantaneous pressure difference between aorta and left ventricle. Pressure half-time is the time required for the maximal pressure gradient, derived by Doppler, to drop by 50%. This index relates inversely with the severity of aortic regurgitation.[67] Flow velocity in the upper descending aorta, recorded from the suprasternal notch, provides additional information in aortic regurgitation by assessing the magnitude of the retrograde diastolic velocity. Table 1.4 lists the Doppler measurements most commonly used and their relation to severity of valvular regurgitation. All of them are subject to technical and measurement errors and thus it is essential that they be obtained by experienced echocardiographers. When properly performed, the results of this integrated analysis can be as accurate as those obtained by angiography with the added advantage that the evaluation can be performed serially.

TABLE 1.4. Doppler Measurements Used in the Evaluation of Valvular Regurgitation, and Their Relation to Severity

Doppler Measurement	Mild (1+)	Moderate (2+)	Moderate to Severe (3+)	Severe (4+)
Mitral regurgitation				
Regurgitant jet area (cm^2)	<2	2–4	5–9	>10
Proximal jet height (mm)	≤5	6–8	9–12	>12
Regurgitant fraction (%)	<20	25–40	41–55	>55
Effective regurgitant orifice area (cm^2)	<0.10	0.10–0.25	0.25–0.35	>0.35
Aortic regurgitation				
Proximal jet height (%)*	≤20	21–50	51–70	>70
Proximal jet area (%)†	<5	6–29	30–60	>60
Regurgitant fraction (%)	<20	25–39	40–55	>55
Pressure half-time (msec)	>600	400–600	200–390	<200

*Expressed as percentage of LV outflow diameter.
†Expressed as percentage of LV outflow area.

Stenotic valvular lesions are quantitated primarily with CW Doppler which allows recording of high flow velocities from which the transvalvular pressure gradient is estimated using the modified Bernoulli equation. In aortic stenosis, the stenotic valve area is derived with the continuity equation. Valve area = the flow passing through the valve, determined by PW, divided by the velocity of the stenotic jet obtained by CW.[68] In mitral stenosis, the valve orifice can be visualized by 2D and its area measured by planimetry.[69] In addition, one can measure pressure half-time as an index of severity and derive the stenotic valve area as 220/pressure half-time,[70] or alternatively, apply the continuity equation.[71] The accuracy of Doppler-derived pressure gradients and stenotic valve areas have been well validated against catheter-derived measurements.[68–73] Nowadays, it is common for patients to undergo the entire valvular evaluation noninvasively utilizing coronary angiography to exclude significant arteriopathy prior to valve repair or replacement. TEE is at times needed whenever the evaluation is inadequate by the transthoracic approach.

Echocardiography with 2D and Doppler is used in patients after valve repair or replacement to assess the functional integrity of the valve and the overall cardiac function. Prosthetic valves as a rule are mildly stenotic and their function is assessed by Doppler as with native valves.[74,75] In some cases of valve regurgitation, particularly in the mitral position, TEE may be needed to enhance sensitivity and to determine the mechanism of regurgitation or obstruction (see Chapter 6).

Myxomatous mitral valve degeneration, also known as mitral valve prolapse (MVP), is one particular lesion that merits individual discussion. This condition is a well-defined clinical entity that, although relatively benign, can be complicated by progressive worsening of mitral regurgitation (MR) or development of acute MR secondary to ruptured chordae tendinea and by endocarditis. In fact, this entity is now the most common cause of mitral regurgitation requiring surgical repair in the United States.[76] In addition, MVP has been associated with cerebral embolic episodes, the pathophysiology of which is not well elucidated.[77] On the other hand, MVP has been frequently blamed as the cause for palpitations, dizziness, and other functional symptoms without proper documentation. Furthermore, this condition has been overdiagnosed by echocardiographers using criteria that are poorly specific. Posterior displacement of the coaptation point of the mitral valve, particularly in the apical views, should not be used alone to diagnose MVP unless it is accompanied by morphologic evidence of valve thickening and redundancy, and/or evidence by Doppler of mitral regurgitation.[77,78]

Evaluation for Endocarditis

The hallmark of infectious endocarditis is the presence of vegetations in the affected valve. These mass-like structures can be visualized with current transthoracic 2D examination in about 50–80% of native valve infections but only in about 20–40% of prosthetic valve infections.[79] Other complications of endocarditis such as abscesses and fistulae are even more difficult to detect. On the other hand, these lesions can all be accurately visualized with TEE even in patients with prosthetic valves.[80,81] TEE has, therefore, become the preferred technique in patients with suspected or proven endocarditis, and will be discussed in more detail in Chapter 6. Any patient with a clinical scenario suspicious of endocarditis should undergo an echocardiographic examination followed by TEE if the former does not provide an adequate positive or negative diagnosis (Table 1.3). The Doppler techniques are essential in these patients to evaluate the severity of valvular regurgitation and localize abnormal fistulae connections.

Evaluation of Intracardiac Masses

Echocardiography is the most commonly used imaging technique for detection and evaluation of intracardiac masses. Most pathologic masses are >1 cm in diameter and thus are readily visualized by 2D unless they are located in a difficult area of the heart to examine, such as in the left atrial appendage. In these instances a TEE examination is indicated. The differential diagnosis of an intracardiac mass seen by ultrasound includes: (1) artifacts (also known as "phantom echoes"), (2) normal structures such as a Chiari network in the right atrium (RA) or a muscle tendon in the LV, (3) thrombi, (4) tumors, and (5) vegetations. Considerable experience is needed to differentiate artifacts and normal variants from pathologic masses. Color flow Doppler may help in detecting vascularity within a mass, such as in some types of atrial myxomas. Currently, echocardiography is often used as the only test to identify intracardiac masses and make therapeutic decisions, including surgical resection. It is therefore crucial that the diagnosis be established with complete certainty.

Echocardiography is limited in its ability to determine the histologic diagnosis of an intracardiac mass. However, at times the location and appearance of the mass may suggest its histologic diagnosis. For instance, a mass attached to an akinetic left ventricular apex is a thrombus until proven otherwise. Likewise, a mass in the left atrium attached to the interatrial septum is most likely a myxoma rather than a thrombus. The clinical scenario may also help in establishing the etiology of a mass, for instance, a mass attached to a valve in a patient with fever is more likely a vegetation than a tumor. The clinical scenarios more frequently associated with intracardiac masses are listed in Table 1.3. However, it is not uncommon for these lesions to be detected as an incidental finding in a study requested for other clinical indications.

Although it is common practice, the routine use of echocardiography in patients with strokes to detect a cardiac source of embolization is not warranted for several reasons. First, with the exception of LV thrombi, other common intracardiac or intravascular sources of embolization (thrombi in the left atrial appendage, complex atheroma in the aorta) are diagnosed better by TEE than by transthoracic echocardiography. Patients likely to have LV thrombi and who are candidates for echocardiographic evaluation are readily recognized by their clinical history and/or electrocardiogram. Second, many patients with strokes have well-established risk factors such as hypertension. Finally, even those with cerebral embolizations often have clinical indications for chronic anticoagulation such as atrial fibrillation, and thus the results of the echocardiographic examination will have little or no impact on patient management. On the other hand, echocardiography may be of diagnostic value in patients with cerebral embolic episodes in whom no clear etiology is elucidated from the standard clinical evaluation.

Evaluation of Pericardial Effusions/Constriction

Detection of pericardial effusion was one of the earliest applications of echocardiography.[1,82] With the current quality of instrumentation, the sensitivity of 2D is nearly 100% with similarly high specificity. Furthermore, echocardiography allows one to define the location and extent of the effusion, grade severity and detect fibrous strands, clots, and other masses within the pericardial space. Increases in intrapericardial pressure induce changes in the mobility of the RV and right atrial free wall as well as respiratory variations in the transmitral velocity by Doppler. Inspiration causes a $\geq 20\%$ drop in E-velocity that recovers with expiration. These changes can assist in the diagnosis of cardiac tamponade.[83–85] However, tamponade is a clinical entity that should be diagnosed at the bedside and not in an echocardiography laboratory. The echo findings are helpful but all of them have sources of false-negative and false-positive results. The clinical situations where echocardiography is frequently used to detect and assess pericardial effusion are listed in Table 1.5.

Constrictive pericarditis can at times be a difficult clinical diagnosis to make. Patients most commonly present with unexplained right heart failure, and the picture may be confused with that of restrictive cardiomyopathy. The 2D/M-mode echo features of constriction are subtle and not very sensitive or specific. Because of the bright reflections that are commonly seen with a normal pericardium, the diagnosis of a thickened pericardium is often not accurate. On the other hand, PW Doppler has been found to be very useful in suggesting the presence of pericardial constriction and distinguishing it from myocardial restriction. With constriction, there is significant respiratory variation of the mitral velocity, similar to that seen with tamponade.[86] In addition, the hepatic vein velocity pattern is distinctly different from that of restrictive cardiomyopathy.[87] In constriction, there is normal ante-

TABLE 1.5. Indications for Echocardiography: Pericardium, Aorta, and Congenital Heart Lesions

Indications	Common Clinical Scenarios

1. Pericardial effusion/constriction
 	
  2D: Diagnosis, assessment of severity, signs of tamponade
  Doppler: Respiratory variation in mitral flow velocity as a sign suggestive of tamponade or constriction
	Recent cardiac surgery with hypotension or dyspnea
	Metastatic cancer with chest pain, hypotension, or dyspnea
	Chest pain suspicious of pericarditis
	Uremic pericarditis
	Unexplained cardiomegaly or pericardial calcification
	Serial evaluation following removal of fluid or medical therapy
	Unexplained right heart failure (constriction)

2. Evaluation of the aorta
  2D: Size aneurysms, dissection
  Doppler: Detection and evaluation of aortic regurgitation
	Murmur of aortic regurgitation
	Chest pain
	Enlarged aorta on chest x-ray
	Marfan's syndrome (or family screening)
	Suspected dissection of the aorta (TEE is better suited than 2D)

3. Congenital heart disease
  2D: Anatomic diagnosis, LV function
  Doppler: Intracardiac shunts, valvular regurgitation, or stenosis
	Heart murmur suggestive of a congenital defect
	Known congenital heart disease
	  a. Evaluation of severity of lesion
	  b. Assessment of cardiac function
	  c. Evaluation after surgical repair

grade systolic flow velocity in the hepatic vein with retrograde late diastolic flow during expiration, while in restriction, antegrade systolic flow is diminished or totally abolished. Differentiation between constriction and restriction can be difficult when patients are in atrial fibrillation or when both conditions coexist in the same patient.

Evaluation of the Aorta

The aortic root and ascending aorta are well visualized by transthoracic 2D echocardiography. In contrast, the arch and descending thoracic aorta are much better seen with TEE, so much so, that the latter procedure is recommended as a primary test in patients with suspected aortic dissection (see Chapter 6). Echocardiography is often the first test to diagnose an aneurysm of the aortic root and/or ascending aorta. Whenever an aneurysm is diagnosed, Doppler should be used to detect aortic regurgitation and assess its severity. Patients frequently present with a murmur of aortic regurgitation, clinical features or family history of Marfan's syndrome, history of chest pain, or abnormal mediastinal silhouette on chest x-Ray (Table 1.5). They may even be detected as an incidental finding on an echocardiogram performed for another clinical reason. Echocardiography is also used to follow the size of an aortic root aneurysm in an asymptomatic patient. Meticulous attention to technical details and expertise are needed in order to obtain reproducible measurements of the aortic root and ascending aorta. When in doubt about these measurements, computerized tomography (CT) or magnetic resonance imaging (MRI) should be obtained, particularly if surgery is being considered purely on the basis of size.

Congenital Heart Disease

Echocardiography is currently the imaging modality of choice for the diagnosis and evaluation of congenital heart lesions (Table 1.5). Color flow and the other Doppler modalities are used to assess intracardiac shunts and valvular lesions. In selected cases, the intravenous injection of agitated saline or 5% dextrose in water is used as an echocardiographic contrast agent to detect right-to-left shunts. Although the majority of patients with congenital heart defects are evaluated by pediatric cardiologists, an increasing number of adults are presenting to the adult cardiologist with previously undetected lesions, such as atrial septal defects (ASD) or Ebstein's anomaly, or with history of surgical "repairs" as children. The latter group frequently presents with residual lesions or complications arising from the surgical procedure. Echocardiography plays a major role in the evaluation of these patients. In selected patients, TEE may be indicated to better visualize a specific lesion such as a sinus venosus ASD. Evaluation of the pulmonary arteries, particularly distal to the main bifurcation, can be difficult by echocardiography even using TEE. These and other complex vascular anomalies can be better visualized using MRI. Invasive cardiac catheterization and angiography are seldom necessary in the adult patient with congenital heart defects except for the evaluation of the coronary arteries.

CONTRAINDICATIONS

Given its noninvasive nature, there are no contraindications to a resting echocardiographic examination. In fact, the test is performed frequently in critically ill patients, a group in whom the results frequently alter their management. The contraindications of stress echocardiography are the same as those of any other stress test; mainly, unstable ischemic syndromes, life-threatening arrhythmias, or contraindications to the use of a particular pharmacologic agent.

ADVANTAGES AND DISADVANTAGES

Echocardiography has several advantages over other imaging techniques. It is performed rapidly with immediate results and is free of harmful effects. The instruments are portable and the cost is relatively less than other techniques such as CT, MRI, or radionuclide studies. Importantly, echocardiography provides accurate results for the majority of the questions asked. It is often the echocardiographer who recommends an alternative test when he/she sees that the echo cannot properly answer the questions addressed by the clinician. For instance, the echocardiographer may suggest an MRI in a patient with features consistent with pericardial constriction in order to accurately measure pericardial thickness. The primary limitation of echocardiography is its dependence on image quality and therefore, on the skills of the sonographer, and importantly on the expertise of the echocardiographer. Even common indications such as evaluation of LV function and regional wall motion are among the most challenging in terms of expertise requirements. A practical disadvantage of echocardiography is that images are currently stored on video tapes and consequently, the quality is degraded when compared to the original image. In addition, the studies are cumbersome to find when multiple patients are stored in one tape and the physicians have to come to the laboratory to see the echo images on their patients. This limitation will hopefully soon be overcome by new developments in digital image storage. Specific limitations relative to individual topics have been discussed.

SPECIAL CONSIDERATIONS

When properly utilized, echocardiography is a very cost-effective diagnostic test that provides results that impact patient care. On the other hand, the test is frequently overused, resulting in an increase expenditure that may not influence the well-being of a patient. The following are examples of uses of echocardiography that have been shown not to be cost-effective.

1. Routine checkup in an asymptomatic patient with no clinical signs of heart disease.
2. Ambulatory patient with recurrent chest pain and without a specific abnormality on physical examination, chest x-Ray, or ECG. While a resting echo is of little benefit, a stress echo is cost-effective.
3. Patients with palpitations without an identified arrhythmia or a specific abnormality on physical examination or ECG.
4. Innocent murmurs in a young asymptomatic patient with no other abnormalities on physical examination, ECG, or chest x-Ray.
5. Elderly patients with strokes in whom anticoagulation is already indicated or who have well-established risk factors for stroke.

FUTURE ADVANCES

The field of ultrasound continues to experience technological advancements that will improve further the diagnostic capabilities of echocardiography. Newer systems are now capable of providing better penetration, higher image resolution, and faster frame rates. The latter is of particular importance when performing color flow Doppler. These systems are increasingly driven by computer processors that allow

TABLE 1.6. New Technological Developments in Echocardiography

Development	Description	Potential Clinical Uses
Doppler tissue imaging	Application of Doppler to record the velocity of moving structures such as myocardium utilizing either spectral or color modalities	Quantitative assessment of regional contraction and relaxation in patients with CAD and other forms of myocardial diseases
Tissue characterization	Quantitative analysis (in decibels) of reflected ultrasound	Differentiate blood from tissue in order to have automated endocardial border recognition
		Automated spectral Doppler quantitation
		Differentiate scar from ischemic and viable myocardium
		Detection of infiltrative cardiomyopathies
		Detection of heart transplant rejection
Three-dimensional reconstruction	Computer reconstruction of three-dimensional real time images from multiple 2D images obtained in a particular sequence	More accurate quantitation of LV volumes and mass
		3D evaluation of valvular lesions, intracardiac masses, and congenital heart defects
		3D reconstruction of myocardial perfusion defects in combination with contrast echocardiography
		3D reconstruction of color flow jets such as in valvular regurgitation
Second harmonic imaging (Contrast echocardiography)	Processing of the returning echoes is designed to preferentially record the energy of frequencies that are harmonics of the resonance frequency of a gas-containing microbubble, in order to enhance visualization of these bubbles.	Assess myocardial perfusion from an intravenous injection of an echo contrast agent
		Improve quantitation of LV function
		Develop new methods to evaluate valvular regurgitation using contrast densitometry

them to improve through software developments and not become obsolescent within a few years. The industry is gradually moving toward digital image storage and transmission that will ultimately eliminate video tapes and facilitate image retrieval and communication with nurses' stations and physicians' offices.

Contrast echocardiography is one of the most promising areas of development in diagnostic ultrasound. Small gas-containing microbubbles act as strong sound reflectors and therefore can be used to image blood flow through cardiac chambers and importantly, through the myocardium.[13,88–90] They can also serve to enhance weak Doppler signals with either spectral or color flow Doppler. Intravenous injection of a contrast agent containing millions of these small microbubbles can pass through the pulmonary capillary bed and appear on the left-sided chambers. The first of these agents, Albunex, has already been approved for clinical use. Albunex consists of air-filled microspheres of human albumin, averaging 4 microns in diameter. This agent is available for enhancement of the LV cavity to better delineate the endocardial borders when assessing LV function and regional wall motion.[91] It can also enhance weak Doppler signals. Although Albunex does not provide adequate myocardial opacification, its recent approval has opened the door to other companies to invest in developing newer agents. Preliminary observations with these new agents in animals are extremely encouraging and raise the realistic expectation that evaluation of myocardial perfusion will be possible in humans. In addition, the ultrasound industry is working on technological developments, such as second harmonic imaging,[92] to facilitate the visualization of these new agents within the myocardium.

Table 1.6 lists the new developments that are becoming available now or in the very near future.

SUMMARY AND CONCLUSIONS

Echocardiography has evolved in 30 years from the limited M-mode technique to a highly sophisticated family of diagnostic modalities with wide clinical applications. It has also become the most utilized noninvasive imaging test in cardiology and thus, a primary contributor to the cost of caring for cardiovascular patients. When ordered properly and performed by competent laboratories, echocardiography can be a very cost-effective test given that it frequently provides definitive diagnostic information and eliminates the need for more expensive tests. The latter statement is particularly true with the addition of TEE in selected clinical conditions as discussed in Chapter 6. The anticipated new developments discussed above are likely to further expand the applications of echocardiography, particularly in patients with ischemic heart disease.

REFERENCES

1. Edler I: The diagnostic use of ultrasound in heart disease. *Acta Med Scand Suppl* 308:332,1955.
2. American College of Cardiology/American Heart Association Guidelines for the clinical application of echocardiography: a report of the American College of Cardiology/American Heart Association Task Force on assessment of diagnostic and therapeutic cardiovascular procedures (subcommittee to develop guidelines for the clinical application of echocardiography). *J Am Coll Cardiol* 16:1505–1528, 1990.

3. Schiller NB, Shah PM, Crawford M, et al: Recommendation for quantitation of the left ventricle by two-dimensional echocardiography. *J Am Soc Echocardiogr* 2:358–367, 1989.

4. Borow KM, Green LH, Mann T, et al: End-systolic volume as a predictor of postoperative left ventricular performance in volume overload from valvular regurgitation. *Am J Med* 68:655–663, 1980.

5. Enriquez-Sarano M, Tajik AJ, Scaff HV, et al: Echocardiographic prediction of left ventricular function after correction of mitral regurgitation: results and clinical implications. *J Am Coll Cardiol* 24:1536–1543, 1994.

6. White HD, Norris RM, Brown MA, et al: Left ventricular end-systolic volume as the major determinant of survival after recovery from myocardial infarction. *Circulation* 76:44–51, 1987.

7. Bonarjee VV, Carstensen S, Caidahl K, et al: Attenuation of left ventricular dilatation after acute myocardial infarction by early initiation of enalapril therapy. CONSENSUS 11 Multi-Echo Study Group. *Am J Cardiol* 72:1004–1009, 1993.

8. Quiñones MA, Waggoner AD, Reduto LA, et al: A new, simplified and accurate method for determining ejection fraction with two-dimensional echocardiography. *Circulation* 64:744–753, 1981.

9. Starling MR, Crawford MH, Sorenson SG, et al: Comparative accuracy of apical biplane cross-sectional echocardiography and gated equilibrium radionuclide angiography for estimating left ventricular size and performance. *Circulation* 63:1075–1084, 1981.

10. Schiller NB, Acquatella H, Ports TA, et al: Left ventricular volume from paired biplane two-dimensional echocardiography. *Circulation* 60:547–555, 1979.

11. Naik MN, Diamond GA, Pai T, et al: Correspondence of left ventricular ejection fraction determinations from two-dimensional echocardiography, radionuclide angiography and contrast echocardiography. *J Am Coll Cardiol* 25:937–942, 1995.

12. Otto CM, Stratton MD, Althouse R, et al: Echocardiographic evaluation of segmental wall motion early and late after thrombolytic therapy in acute myocardial infarction: the Western Washington Tissue Plasminogen Activator Emergency Room Trial. *Am J Cardiol* 65:132–138, 1990.

13. Ito H, Tomooka T, Sakai N, et al: Lack of myocardial perfusion immediately after successful thrombolysis: a predictor of poor recovery of left ventricular function in anterior myocardial infarction. *Circulation* 85:1699–1705, 1992.

14. Berning J, Steensgaard-Hansen F: Early estimation of risk by echocardiographic determination of wall motion index in an unselected population with acute myocardial infarction. *Am J Cardiol* 65:567–576, 1990.

15. Nishimura RA, Tajik AJ, Shub C, et al: Role of two-dimensional echocardiography in the prediction of in-hospital complications after acute myocardial infarction. *J Am Coll Cardiol* 4:1080–1087, 1984.

16. VanReet R, Quiñones MA, Poliner LA, et al: Comparison of two-dimensional echocardiography with gated radionuclide ventriculography in the evaluation of global and regional left ventricular function in acute myocardial infarction. *J Am Coll Cardiol* 3:243–252, 1984.

17. Candell-Riera J, Permanyer-Miralda G, Castell J, et al: Uncomplicated first myocardial infarction: strategy for comprehensive prognostic studies. *J Am Coll Cardiol* 18:1207–1219, 1991.

18. Levy D, Garrison RJ, Savage DD, et al: Prognostic implication of echocardiographically determined left ventricular mass in the Framingham heart study. *N Engl J Med* 322:1561–1566, 1990.

19. Sullivan JM, Vander Zwaag RV, el-Zeky F, et al: Left ventricular hypertrophy: effect on survival. *J Am Coll Cardiol* 22:508–513, 1993.

20. Levy D, Salomon M, D'Agostino RB, et al: Prognostic implications of baseline electro-cardiographic features and their serial changes in subjects with left ventricular hypertro-phy. *Circulation* 90:1786–1793, 1994.

21. Casale PN, Devereux RB, Milner M, et al: Value of echocardiographic measurement of left ventricular mass in predicting cardiovascular morbid events in hypertensive men. *Ann Intern Med* 105:173–178, 1986.

22. Cooper RS, Simmons BE, Castaner A, et al: Left ventricular hypertrophy is associated with worse survival independent of ventricular function and number or coronary arteries severely narrowed. *Am J Cardiol* 65:441–445, 1990.

23. Woythaler JN, Singer SL, Kwan OL, et al: Accuracy of echocardiography versus elec-trocardiography in detecting left ventricular hypertrophy: comparison with post-mortem mass measurements. *J Am Coll Cardiol* 2:305–311, 1983.

24. Reichek N, Devereux RB: Left ventricular hypertrophy: relationship of anatomic, echocardiographic and electrocardiographic findings. *Circulation* 63:1391–1398, 1981.

25. Triulzi M, Gillam LD, Gentile F, et al: Normal adult cross-sectional echocardiographic val-ues: linear dimensions and chamber areas. *Echocardiography* 1:403–426, 1984.

26. Lewis JF, Kuo LC, Nelson JG, et al: Pulsed Doppler echocardiographic determination of stroke volume and cardiac output: clinical validation of two new methods using the api-cal window. *Circulation* 70:425–431, 1984.

27. Rakowski H, Sasson Z, Wile ED: Echocardiographic and Doppler assessment of hyper-trophic cardiomyopathy. *J Am Soc Echocardiogr* 1:31–47, 1988.

28. Currie PJ, Seward JB, Chan KL, et al: Continuous wave Doppler determination of right ventricular pressure: a simultaneous Doppler-catheterization study in 127 patients. *J Am Coll Cardiol* 6:750–756, 1985.

29. Kircher BS, Himelman RB, Schiller NB: Noninvasive estimation of right atrial pressure from the inspiratory collapse of the inferior vena cava. *Am J Cardiol* 66:493–496, 1990.

30. Naqueh SF, Kopelen HA, Zoghbi WA: Relation of mean right atrial pressure to echocar-diographic and Doppler parameters of right atrial and right ventricular function. *Circu-lation* 93:1160–1169, 1996.

31. Himelman RB, Stulbarg M, Kircher B, et al: Noninvasive evaluation of pulmonary artery pressure during exercise by saline-enhanced Doppler echocardiography in chronic pul-monary disease. *Circulation* 79:863–871, 1989.

32. Appleton CP, Hartle LK, Popp RL. Relation of transmitral flow velocity patterns to left ventricular diastolic function. New insights from a combined hemodynamic and Doppler echocardiographic study. *J Am Coll Cardiol* 12:426–440, 1988.

33. Nishimura RA, Abel MD, Hatle LK, et al: Relation of pulmonary vein to mitral flow veloc-ities by transesophageal Doppler echocardiography. Effect of different loading condi-tions. *Circulation* 81:1488–1497, 1990.

34. Nishimura RA, Abel MD, Hatle LK, et al: Assessment of diastolic function of the heart: background and current applications of Doppler echocardiography. Part II. Clinical stud-ies. *Mayo Clin Proc* 64:181–204, 1989.

35. Appleton CP, Galloway JM, Gonzalez MS, et al: Estimation of left ventricular filling pres-sures using two-dimensional and Doppler echocardiography in adult patients with cardiac disease. *J Am Coll Cardiol* 22:1971–1982, 1993.

36. Kuercherer HF, Muhiudeen IA, Kusumoto FM, et al: Estimation of mean left atrial pressure from transesophageal pulsed Doppler echocardiography of pulmonary venous flow. *Circulation* 82:1127–1139, 1990.

37. Rossvoll O, Hatle LK: Pulmonary venous flow velocities recorded by transthoracic Doppler ultrasound: relation to left ventricular diastolic pressures. *J Am Coll Cardiol* 21:1687–1696, 1993.

38. Mulvagh S, Quiñones MA, Kleiman NS, et al: Estimation of left ventricular end-diastolic pressure from Doppler transmitral flow velocity in cardiac patients independent of systolic performance. *J Am Coll Cardiol* 20:112–119, 1992.

39. Nagueh SF, Kopelen HA, Zoghbi WA: Feasibility and accuracy of Doppler echocardiographic estimation of pulmonary artery occlusive pressure in the intensive care unit. *Am J Cardiol* 75:1256–1262, 1995.

40. Gross GJ, Warltier DC: Coronary steal in four models of single or multiple vessel obstruction in dogs. *Am J Cardiol* 48:84–91, 1981.

41. Limacher MC, Quiñones MA, Poline LS, et al: Detection of coronary artery disease with exercise two-dimensional echocardiography. Description of a clinically applicable method and comparison with radionuclide ventriculography. *Circulation* 67:1211–1218, 1983.

42. Armstrong WF, O'Donnell J, Ryan T, et al: Effect of prior myocardial infarction and extent and location of coronary disease on accuracy of exercise echocardiography. *J Am Coll Cardiol* 10:531–538, 1987.

43. Quiñones MA, Verani MS, Haichin RN, et al: Exercise echocardiography versus thallium-201 single photon emission computed tomography in the evaluation of coronary artery disease: analysis of 292 patients. *Circulation* 85:1026–1031, 1992.

44. Hecht HA, DeBord L, Shaw R: Supine bicycle stress echocardiography versus tomographic thallium-201 exercise imaging for the detection of coronary artery disease. *J Am Soc Echocardiogr* 6:177–185, 1993.

45. Sawada SG, Segar DS, Ryan T, et al: Echocardiographic detection of coronary artery disease during dobutamine infusion. *Circulation* 83:1605–1614, 1991.

46. Cohen JL, Green TO, Ottenweller J, et al: Dobutamine digital echocardiography for detecting coronary artery disease. *Am J Cardiol* 67:1311–1318, 1991.

47. Beleslin BD, Ostojic M, Stepanovic J, et al: Stress echocardiography in the detection of myocardial ischemia. Head-to-head comparison of exercise, dobutamine, and dipyridamole tests. *Circulation* 90:1168–1176, 1994.

48. Marcovitz PA, Armstrong WF: Accuracy of dobutamine stress echocardiography in detecting coronary artery disease. *Am J Cardiol* 69:1269–1273, 1992.

49. Zoghbi WA, Cheirif J, Kleiman NS, et al: Diagnosis of ischemic heart disease using adenosine echocardiography. *J Am Coll Cardiol* 18:1271–1279, 1991.

50. Picano E, Pingitore A, Conti U, et al: Enhanced sensitivity for detection of coronary artery disease by addition of atropine to dipyridamole echocardiography. *Eur Heart J* 14:1216–1222, 1993.

51. Jaarsma W, Visser CA, Funke Kupper AJ, et al: Usefulness of two-dimensional exercise echocardiography shortly after myocardial infarction. *Am J Cardiol* 57:86–90, 1986.

52. Ryan T, Armstrong WF, O'Donnell JA, et al: Risk stratification after acute myocardial infarction by means of exercise two-dimensional echocardiography. *Am Heart J* 114:1305–1316, 1987.

53. Severi S, Picano E, Michelassi C, et al: Diagnostic and prognostic value of dipyridamole

echocardiography in patients with suspected coronary artery disease. Comparison with exercise electrocardiography. *Circulation* 89:1160–1173, 1994.

54. Krivokapich J, Child JS, Gerber R, et al: Prognostic usefulness of positive or negative exercise stress echocardiography for predicting coronary events in ensuing twelve months. *Am J Cardiol* 71:646–651, 1993.

55. Davila-Roman VG, Waggoner AD, Sicard GA, et al: Dobutamine stress echocardiography predicts surgical outcome in patients with an aortic aneurysm and peripheral vascular disease. *J Am Coll Cardiol* 21:957–963, 1993.

56. Olmos LI, Gordon RJ, Dakik H, et al: Long term prognostic value of exercise echocardiography compared to thallium-201 perfusion imaging, electrocardiographic and clinical variables in patients evaluated for coronary artery disease (abstract). *Circulation* 92:1–411, 1995.

57. La Canna G, Alfiere O, Giubbini R, et al: Echocardiography during infusion of dobutamine for identification of reversible dysfunction in patients with chronic coronary artery disease. *J Am Coll Cardiol* 23:617–626, 1994.

58. Perrone-Filardi P, Pace L, Prastaro M, et al: Dobutamine echocardiography predicts improvement of hypoperfused dysfunctional myocardium after revascularization in patients with coronary artery disease. *Circulation* 91:2556–2565, 1995.

59. Afridi I, Kleiman NS, Raizner AE, et al: Dobutamine echocardiography in myocardial hibernation. Optimal dose and accuracy in predicting recovery of ventricular function coronary angioplasty. *Circulation* 91:663–670, 1995.

60. Marwick T, Willemart B, D'Hondt AM, et al: Selection of the optimal nonexercise stress for the evaluation of ischemic regional myocardial dysfunction and malperfusion. Comparison of dobutamine and adenosine using echocardiography and ^{99m}Tc-MIBI single photon emission computed tomography. *Circulation* 87:345–354, 1993.

61. Helmcke F, Nanda NC, Hsiung MC, et al: Color Doppler assessment of mitral regurgitation with orthogonal planes. *Circulation* 85:1248–1253, 1992.

62. Chen C, Thomas JD, Anconina J, et al: Impact of impinging wall jet on color Doppler quantification of mitral regurgitation. *Circulation* 84:712–720, 1991.

63. Perry GL, Helmcke F, Nanda NC, et al: Evaluation of aortic insufficiency by Doppler color flow mapping. *J Am Coll Cardiol* 9:952–959, 1987.

64. Mele D, Vandervoort P, Palacios I, et al: Proximal jet size by Doppler color flow mapping predicts severity of mitral regurgitation: clinical studies. *Circulation* 91:746–754, 1995.

65. Enriquez-Sarano M, Miller FA, Hayes SN, et al: Effective mitral regurgitant orifice area: clinical use and pitfalls of the proximal isovelocity surface area method. *J Am Coll Cardiol* 25:703–709, 1995.

66. Rokey R, Sterling LL, Zoghbi WA, et al: Determination of regurgitant fraction in isolated mitral or aortic regurgitation by pulsed-Doppler two-dimensional echocardiography. *J Am Coll Cardiol* 7:1273–1278, 1986.

67. Teague SM, Heinsimer JA, Anderson JL, et al: Quantification of aortic regurgitation utilizing continuous wave Doppler ultrasound. *J Am Coll Cardiol* 8:592–599, 1986.

68. Zoghbi WA, Farmer KL, Soto JG, et al: Accurate noninvasive quantification of stenotic aortic valve area by Doppler echocardiography. *Circulation* 73:452–459, 1986.

69. Martin RP, Rakowski H, Kleiman JH, et al: Reliability and reproducibility of two-dimensional echocardiograph measurement of the stenotic mitral valve orifice area. *Am J Cardiol* 43:560–568, 1979.

70. Stamm RB, Martin RP: Quantification of pressure gradients across stenotic valves by Doppler ultrasound. *J Am Coll Cardiol* 2:707–718, 1983.

71. Nakatani S, Masuyama T, Kodama K, et al: Value and limitations of Doppler echocardiography in the quantification of stenotic mitral valve area: comparison of the pressure half-time and continuity equation methods. *Circulation* 77:78–85, 1988.

72. Galan A, Zoghbi WA, Quiñones MA: Determination of severity of valvular aortic stenosis by Doppler echocardiography and relation of findings to clinical outcome and agreement to hemodynamics determined at cardiac catheterization. *Am J Cardiol* 67:1007–1012, 1991.

73. Oh JK, Taliercio CP, Holmes DR Jr, et al: Prediction of the severity of aortic stenosis by Doppler aortic valve area determination: prospective Doppler catheterization correlation in 100 patients. *J Am Coll Cardiol* 11:1227–1234, 1988.

74. Reisner SA, Meltzer RS: Normal values of prosthetic valve Doppler echocardiographic parameters. *J Am Soc Echocardiogr* 1:201–210, 1988.

75. Chafizadeh ER, Zoghbi WA: Doppler echocardiographic assessment of the St. Jude medical prosthetic valve in the aortic position using the continuity equation. *Circulation* 83:213–223, 1991.

76. Waller BF, Morrow AG, Maron BJ, et al: Etiology of clinically isolated, severe, chronic pure mitral regurgitation: analysis of 97 patients over 30 years of age having mitral valve replacement. *Am Heart J* 104:276, 1982.

77. Nishimura RA, McGoon MD, Shub C, et al: Echocardiographically documented mitral valve prolapse: long-term follow-up of 237 patients. *N Engl J Med* 313:1305–1309, 1985.

78. Levine RA, Stathogiannis E, Newell JB, et al: Reconsideration of echocardiographic standards for mitral valve prolapse: lack of association between leaflet displacement isolated to the apical four-chamber view and independent echocardiographic evidence of abnormality. *J Am Coll Cardiol* 11:1010–1019, 1988.

79. Jaffe WM, Morgan DE, Pearlman AS, et al: Infective endocarditis, 1983–1988: echocardiographic findings and factors influencing morbidity and mortality. *J Am Coll Cardiol* 15:1227–1233, 1990.

80. Daniel WG, Mugge A, Grote J, et al: Evaluation of endocarditis and its complications by biplane and multiplane transesophageal echocardiography. *Am J Card Imaging* 9:100–105, 1995.

81. Lowry RW, Zoghbi WA, Baker WB, et al: Clinical impact of transesophagel echocardiography in the diagnosis and management of infective endocarditis: significance of negative findings. *Am J Cardiol* 73:1089–1091, 1994.

82. Feigenbaum H, Waldhaussen JA, Hyde LP: Ultrasound diagnosis of pericardial effusion. *JAMA* 191:711–714, 1965.

83. Schiller NB, Botvinick EH: Right ventricular compression as a sign of cardiac tamponade. *Circulation* 56:774–789, 1977.

84. Kronzon I, Cohen ML, Winer HE: Diastolic atrial compression: a sensitive echocardiographic sign of cardiac tamponade. *J Am Coll Cardiol* 2:770–775, 1983.

85. Appleton CP, Hatle LK, Popp RL: Cardiac tamponade and pericardial effusion: respiratory variation in transvalvular flow velocities studied by Doppler echocardiography. *J Am Coll Cardiol* 11:1020–1030, 1988.

86. Hatle KL, Appleton CP, Popp RL. Differentiation of constrictive pericarditis and restrictive cardiomyopathy by Doppler echocardiography. *Circulation* 79:357–370, 1989.

87. Oh JK, Hatle LK, Seward JB, et al: Diagnostic role of Doppler echocardiography in constrictive pericarditis. *J Am Coll Cardiol* 23:154–162, 1994.

88. Cheirif J, Zoghbi WA, Raizner AE, et al: Assessment of myocardial perfusion in man by contrast echocardiography. Phase I. Evaluation of regional coronary reserve by peak contrast intensity. *J Am Coll Cardiol* 11:735–743, 1988.

89. Sabia PJ, Powers ER, Jayaweera AR, et al: Functional significance of collateral blood flow in patients with recent acute myocardial infarction. A study using myocardial contrast echocardiography. *Circulation* 85:2080–2089, 1992.

90. Sabia PJ, Powers ER, Ragosta M, et al: An association between collateral blood flow and myocardial viability in patients with recent myocardial infarction. *N Engl J Med* 327:1825–1831, 1992.

91. Feinstein SB, Cheirif BJ, TenCate FJ, et al: Safety and efficacy of a new transpulmonary ultrasound contrast agent: initial multicenter clinical results. *J Am Coll Cardiol* 16:316–324, 1990.

92. Porter TR, Xie F: Transient myocardial contrast after initial exposure to diagnostic ultrasound pressures with minute doses of intravenously injected microbubbles: demonstration and potential mechanisms. *Circulation* 92:2391–2395, 1995.

─ 2 ─

Nuclear Cardiology Testing

Mario S. Verani, M.D.

In the last two decades nuclear cardiology has flourished and made a claim as a sophisticated, clinically relevant subspecialty. In 1993, the creation of the American Society of Nuclear Cardiology and the implementation of its flagship journal, The *Journal of Nuclear Cardiology*, have given further recognition to this hybrid subspecialty, where knowledge of nuclear physics, instrumentation, cardiology, and computer sciences blend together.

Nuclear cardiology stands out among all the cardiology subspecialties as the one that lends itself best to the use of computer quantification of biologic phenomena. In fact, all of the currently available nuclear cardiology procedures require a computer for acquisition, processing, and quantification. The importance of the electronics and computerization in nuclear cardiology becomes obvious when one realizes that only 1 out of every 3 or 5 photons emitted during the decay of thallium-201 in the left ventricular wall can successfully cross the path from the heart to the gamma camera detector, the remaining being absorbed in the thoracic tissue layers. Thus, computer techniques are pivotal in the transformation of tiny physical phenomena into information that can be visualized and quantified.

DESCRIPTION OF TECHNIQUES

Although nuclear cardiology procedures have been used in the evaluation of a broad spectrum of cardiac pathologies, ranging from intracardiac shunts, to valvular insufficiencies and even pericardial effusions, the two most important contributions of

33

nuclear cardiology in the management of cardiac diseases are the assessment of myocardial blood flow with myocardial perfusion imaging and of ventricular function with radionuclide angiography. Consequently, only these topics will be discussed in this review.

Myocardial Perfusion Imaging: The Paradigm of Noninvasive Determination of Myocardial Blood Flow

Developmental Perspectives

Although myocardial perfusion imaging had been tried with rubidium-82 and potassium-43 in the early 1970s, it was only with the cyclotron-production of the man-made radionuclide thallium-201 in 1973 that perfusion imaging really took off. In the 1970s and early 1980s, myocardial perfusion imaging became increasingly popular throughout the world, using planar imaging. Despite the limitations of planar techniques, which could only display the left ventricular myocardium in 3 or 4 projections, always hampered by a substantial overlap of the different myocardial regions, perfusion imaging became a well-validated, useful diagnostic tool. The advent of single-photon emission computed tomography (SPECT) in the early 1980s was instrumental in further refining and expanding the clinical indications of myocardial perfusion scintigraphy.

Technical Considerations

Myocardial perfusion imaging is performed after the injection of a tracer such as thallium-201 or one of the technetium-labeled compounds (sestamibi, tetrofosmine, or teboroxime are all currently FDA-approved for this purpose). Thallium is usually injected during exercise or pharmacologic stress and images are acquired shortly after and then repeated 4 hr later, to assess for redistribution (filling-in of the stress-induced defects). When one of the technetium-99m-labeled compounds is used, it is necessary to inject the tracer separately during stress and at rest, because redistribution is less complete than that which occurs with thallium-201. In the author's laboratory, the stress images are performed first and only when they are abnormal or borderline do the patients undergo rest or redistribution imaging. A further difference among the tracers is that with thallium-201 image acquisition starts within 5 or 10 min of the injection, whereas with sestamibi and tetrofosmin imaging starts 15 to 30 min or later after the injection (this is because of the initially high liver uptake, which clears over time). With teboroxime the images must be initiated within 1 or 2 min of the injection, due to the rapid myocardial clearance of this tracer.

Because the myocardial blood flow and its surrogate, myocardial perfusion images, may be entirely normal at rest despite the presence of significant coronary stenosis, perfusion imaging is often performed during some type of stress, that will bring about a heterogeneous myocardial blood flow distribution. The ubiquitous phenomenon of normal myocardial blood flow at rest, in spite of even severe coronary stenosis, deserves further discussion. In normal individuals, there is a native coronary flow reserve, which in simple terms can be defined as the ability of the coronary arteries to adjust their flow in order to match the myocardial oxygen demands. Thus, during exercise an increased myocardial oxygen demand is satisfied by vasodilation of the coronary arterioles, which allows an increase in coronary blood flow. During exercise, this increase in flow is of the order of 2 or 3 times the baseline resting flow. The maximal coronary flow reserve can be elicited by potent coronary vasodilators such as adenosine, adenosine 5′-triphosphate (ATP), or dipyridamole, which will produce a 4- or 5-fold increase in coronary blood flow. In normal subjects, this increase in flow is homogeneous throughout the left ventricle, in such a manner that if a radionuclide tracer is injected during stress one would see a normal, homogeneous tracer distribution across the myocardium.

When a coronary stenosis is present, the maximal coronary flow reserve will be reduced in direct proportion to the severity of the stenosis. For example, in the resting state even a stenosis of, say, 80% of the luminal diameter may not be sufficient to reduce the resting flow, because as the coronary stenosis progresses, the coronary arterioles distal to the obstruction will dilate, thereby maintaining the resting blood flow within normal limits. This, however, occurs at expense of the coronary flow reserve, which will limit the ability to further increase the flow during stress. In the hypothetical situation of an 80% coronary stenosis, although flow and perfusion may be normal at rest, during stress the flow will increase normally through the normal coronary arteries, but will increase less (or not at all) in the vessel with a high-grade stenosis. Injection of a tracer at that point will show a heterogeneous perfusion, with normal tracer uptake in the normal vascular territories and comparatively less uptake in the vascular territory supplied by the artery with coronary stenosis. Gould et al., in a series of now classical experimental and clinical studies, demonstrated that the maximal coronary flow reserve begins to be impinged upon when there is a 40% to 50% coronary stenosis and it will be abolished when a very severe stenosis is present (e.g., >80%).[1,2]

In a patient with such severe coronary stenosis, the resting blood flow may be decreased, leading to resting perfusion abnormalities. A resting perfusion abnormality will also be present in patients with recent or old myocardial infarction or scarring. As discussed below, there are ways to differentiate resting perfusion abnormalities that are due to low flow from those due to previous myocardial infarction and scarring.

Myocardial Perfusion Imaging during Stress

Exercise is the most often used stress to elicit perfusion heterogeneities that can be mapped during perfusion scintigraphy. Because exercise is often insufficient to elicit the maximal coronary flow reserve, it is important to emphasize that one should always strive for a maximal test if one is attempting to demonstrate the effects of coronary stenoses on myocardial perfusion. A submaximal exercise test may not be sufficient to provoke enough disparity in the coronary flow among different territories to produce an abnormal scan.

The sensitivity and specificity of thallium-201 SPECT imaging during exercise vary considerably, depending on the interaction of factors such as frequency of maximal versus submaximal tests, presence of anti-ischemic medications, prior occurrence of myocardial infarction, multivessel versus single-vessel disease, severity of individual stenosis, and use of qualitative versus quantitative analysis. A survey of many published studies has shown a sensitivity of 90% and specificity of 70%.[3,4]

The corollary of these figures is that approximately 10% of coronary stenosis will be missed, whereas as many as 30% of patients with a positive test will not have angiographically demonstrable significant stenosis. These numbers, no doubt, have been used by many cardiologists to attempt to justify coronary angiography in all patients with suspected coronary artery disease. However, another interpretation, which is supported by a large number of clinical studies, is that patients with angiographic coronary stenosis and normal perfusion images either have no demonstrable perfusion abnormalities or they are so minute as to go undetected by the current techniques. In any case, many studies have firmly documented that patients with normal perfusion images during stress have an excellent prognosis and an extremely low likelihood of developing cardiac events in the ensuing years.[5] This is true whether or not coronary stenoses are present.

The unexpected high rate of false-positive studies can be explained on the basis of two different mechanisms. One mechanism is based on technical considerations. Photon attenuation can be unusually severe in some patients, thereby creating attenuation artifacts that can be mistaken for true myocardial hypoperfusion. In addition, inadequate quality control may also create artifacts due to patient motion during imaging, inadequate detector uniformity or sensitivity, incorrect axis of rotation, and other technical reasons which may create certain artifacts that can mimic true perfusion defects. The second reason that may explain a low specificity in some reports is the so called "post-test referral bias,"[6] which is based on the premise that patients with an abnormal perfusion scan are preferentially referred to coronary angiography, whereas those with normal scans usually do not undergo coronary angiography. Recent evidence from several laboratories[7,8] indeed suggests that only a minute fraction (a few percentage points) of patients with a normal scan ever undergo coronary angiography, whereas those with an abnormal scan have a much higher likelihood of undergoing coronary angiography. This phenomenon will produce an artificially high number of patients with normal coronary arteries but an abnormal scan, since the abnormal scan was often the reason for undergoing the coronary angiograms.

Recent developments in photon attenuation correction have been quite encouraging and should reduce the number of false-positive images due to photon attenuation, which is probably the main reason for false-positive defects. An example of images with and without attenuation correction is shown in Figure 2.1. As can be appreciated, in the images without attenuation correction in this patient with large breasts, an apparent defect is obvious in the anterior wall of the left ventricle. After attenuation correction, the defect disappears.

Although the newer technetium-99m-labeled myocardial perfusion tracers were developed with the expectation that they might further improve sensitivity and specificity, since ^{99m}Tc offers improved physical properties over thallium-201 (such as a higher photon energy, less attenuation, and higher dosimetry), in practice, only a marginal improvement in overall diagnostic accuracy can be expected with the technetium agents (sestamibi and tetrofosmin).[3,9,10] This may be because despite all the advantages of the ^{99m}Tc-labeled tracers over thallium, they also share a common limitation, namely, a reduced myocardial extraction in comparison with thallium-201 (with the exception of ^{99m}Tc teboroxime, which has a high extraction fraction but a myocardial clearance too rapid to be clinically useful). Nevertheless, the ^{99m}Tc tracers represent a clear advantage over thallium-201 in large, obese patients or in

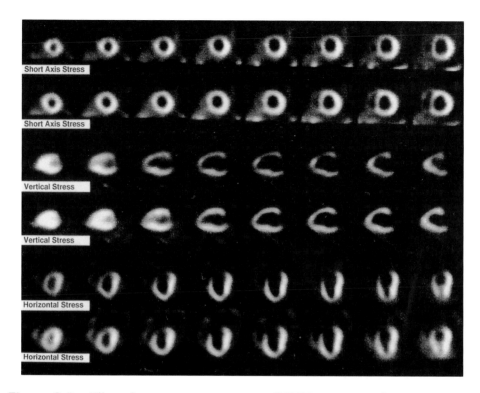

Short Axis Stress

Short Axis Stress

Vertical Stress

Vertical Stress

Horizontal Stress

Horizontal Stress

Figure 2.1. Effect of attenuation correction on SPECT imaging. In this patient, breast shadow mimics a defect in the anterior wall of the left ventricle, which is no longer present after attenuation correction.

women with breast attenuation, in whom the quality of the images is often suboptimal with thallium-201.

Indications and Uses

As shown in Table 2.1, the most important applications of myocardial scintigraphy can be grouped into five broad categories: (1) diagnosis of coronary artery disease (CAD); (2) evaluation of the functional significance of coronary stenosis; (3) evaluation of therapeutic interventions; (4) risk stratification; and (5) assessment of myocardial viability. Detailed discussion of all these topics has been reported recently.[3,9–14] Most of the time the tests are done in patients with various types of chest pains, more or less suggestive of CAD. The tests are usually done during stress (either exercise or pharmacologic stress). A sestamibi perfusion scan has been increasingly used at rest in patients who present to the emergency room with resting chest pains.[15,16] At other times, patients are referred for perfusion imaging because of abnormalities observed on a resting ECG or exercise ECG in patients who do not have angina.

It is controversial whether a patient without symptoms should undergo any stress testing at all. However, middle-aged patients with two or more risk factors for CAD may well benefit from stress perfusion imaging to uncover CAD before the onset of symptoms. This is particularly true with patients who have diabetes.

TABLE 2.1.   Indications for Myocardial Perfusion Imaging

Diagnosis of CAD
   In patients with chest pain syndrome
   In asymptomatic patients with abnormal resting ECG
   In asymptomatic patients with risk factors for CAD
   In patients with an abnormal exercise ECG test
   In patients with coronary stenosis of indeterminate physiologic significance
   Surveillance after orthotopic heart transplant
Evaluation of Functional Significance of Coronary Stenosis
   Before and after percutaneous transluminal coronary angioplasty or coronary artery
      bypass graft surgery
   Before valve surgery
Evaluation of Therapeutic Interventions
   Percutaneous transluminal coronary angioplasty
   Coronary artery bypass graft surgery
   Thrombolytic therapy for acute myocardial infarction
   Anti-ischemic medical therapy
Risk Stratification
   In patients with stable or unstable angina
   In patients with documented CAD without angina
   Postmyocardial infarction
   Before noncardiac surgeries
   In patients with hypertrophic cardiomyopathy
Assessment of Myocardial Viability
   SPECT
   PET

Abbreviations: CAD = coronary artery disease; PET = positron emission tomography; SPECT = single-photon emission computed tomography.

Myocardial perfusion imaging during stress is also theoretically attractive in the surveillance of transplant arteriopathy in patients after an orthotopic heart transplant. However, the ultimate role of perfusion imaging and which kind of stress would be preferable in these patients are not clear at the present time.

Evaluation of the Functional Significance of Coronary Stenosis

In many busy nuclear cardiology laboratories, perhaps 20% to 30% of all perfusion scans are done *after* coronary angiography. This is so because often cardiologists seek to assess the functional significance of coronary stenosis of indeterminate clinical significance. This is particularly true for stenoses of moderate severity (i.e., those between 50% and 70%). A perfusion defect in the territory perfused by one such artery indicates that the lesion is indeed significant, whereas the absence of a perfusion defect at maximal stress suggests the lesion is not functionally significant.

Other times, one questions which one of several lesions is the "culprit," that is, the one responsible for causing myocardial ischemia corresponding to clinical symptoms. This is particularly important in the planning of revascularization procedures in patients with multivessel CAD.

Myocardial perfusion scintigraphy may also afford an excellent means to document the presence of myocardial ischemia in patients with coronary spasm, who may not have fixed lesions observed on coronary angiography. Our group has demonstrated the value of perfusion scintigraphy in such cases in terms of documenting the presence of myocardial ischemia, localizing the area with coronary spasm, and ensuring abolition of myocardial ischemia after appropriate antispasm therapy.[17,18] Figure 2.2 shows an example of a patient with severe exertional angina who had only insignificant lesions by coronary angiography. In this patient, perfusion imaging uncovered extensive myocardial ischemia during exertion before therapy and complete abolition of ischemia after appropriate therapy.

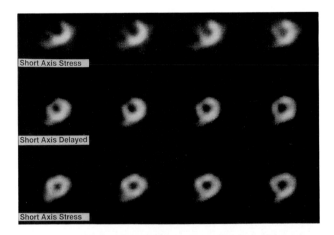

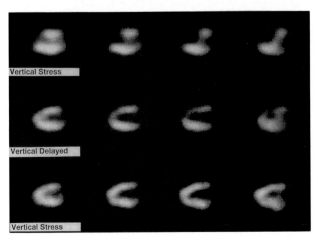

Figure 2.2. A 57-yr-old female patient with typical exertional angina but only "insignificant" plaquing observed in the left anterior descending artery. The Tl-201 SPECT images showed severe anterior septal and apical defects during exercise (*top row*), which filled-in the 4-hr redistribution (*middle row*) images. During exercise, the ECG showed ST-segment elevation in V1–V4. After treatment with a calcium antagonist, the exercise study was entirely normal (*bottom row*). The clinical diagnosis was exercise-induced coronary artery spasm.

At other times, perfusion scintigraphy is called upon to establish the functional significance of coronary restenosis after angioplasty or stents and after coronary artery bypass graft surgery.

Evaluation of Therapeutic Intervention

Myocardial perfusion scintigraphy is an excellent technique to document improvement of myocardial perfusion after coronary angioplasty or coronary artery bypass graft surgery. Although there is no uniform agreement on what is the best timing for perfusion scintigraphy after those interventions, the majority of the improvement in perfusion observed after angioplasty can be documented early after the intervention. It appears prudent to wait approximately 2 wk to perform a stress perfusion study, to avoid the dubious criticism that normal coronary flow dynamics early after angioplasty may possibly account for some defects early on, although this is not very well documented.[19] Our own experience has suggested that transient perfusion defects observed early after angioplasty are not usually false-positives, but rather caused by myocardial hypoperfusion and are indeed associated with a high recurrence rate of angina and coronary stenosis, whereas freedom from perfusion defects early on suggests a persistently high patency rate.[20] In patients with recurrent symptoms, perfusion scintigraphy should be done and will be effective in documenting restenosis and selecting patients who will need repeat coronary angiography and/or additional intervention.

In patients after coronary artery bypass graft surgery, myocardial perfusion scintigraphy is also a powerful technique to demonstrate the improved myocardial perfusion as well as graft patency early and late after bypass graft surgery.[21] Figure 2.3 shows an example of a patient who underwent coronary angioplasty with initial improvement, followed by restenosis and recurrence of symptoms; eventually, coronary stenting led to long-term symptom relief and normalization of the perfusion pattern.

Myocardial perfusion scintigraphy is probably underutilized in the assessment of therapeutic benefits after medical therapy. Our group has recently demonstrated that substantial improvement in myocardial perfusion can be seen following traditional anti-ischemic therapy.[22,23]

As demonstrated in the laboratory animal on an occlusion–reperfusion model[24] and subsequently in patients undergoing thrombolytic therapy or primary angioplasty,[25–27] 99mTc sestamibi SPECT affords an excellent means to assess myocardial salvage following coronary reperfusion. Thallium-201 SPECT imaging also allows accurate quantification of infarct size,[28,29] but is not as useful as sestamibi to demonstrate myocardial salvage after thrombolysis.

Risk Stratification

The prognostic value of stress perfusion scintigraphy has been very well documented in recent years.[3,14] In general, multiple areas of perfusion abnormality, defect reversibility, increased thallium lung uptake during stress, and transient cavity dilatation during stress are powerful markers of high likelihood for cardiac events.[3,14,30,31] More recently, the ability to quantify the extent of myocardial perfusion abnormalities has further refined the value of perfusion scintigraphy.

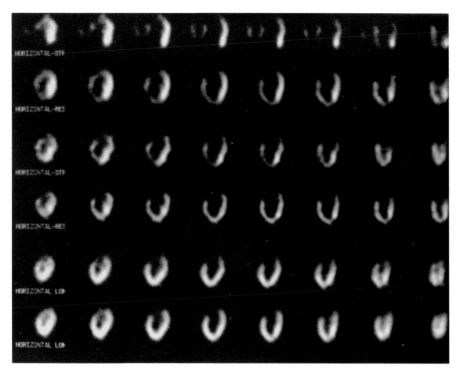

Figure 2.3.   Patient with large anterior, apical, inferior, and septal defects in the exercise images (*top row*) which largely filled-in 4 hr later (*second row from the top*). After angioplasty of the left anterior descending and circumflex arteries there is improved perfusion with a residual defect in the anteroapical region (*third and fourth rows from the top*). After stenting of the left anterior descending artery, the scan is essentially normal (*bottom two rows*). Only the stress-redistribution horizontal long axis images are depicted, before and after angioplasty and after stenting.

Iskandrian and coworkers have demonstrated that perfusion defect sizes involving ≥15% of the left ventricle during stress carry a poor prognosis, whereas perfusion defects involving <15% define a group of patients with a much more benign prognosis. In fact, SPECT may be a more powerful determinant of prognosis than the coronary angiographic findings[32] and further enhances the ability to correctly prognosticate, even in patients with known coronary anatomy.

The prognostic value of perfusion scintigraphy has been equally well demonstrated for a broad spectrum of ischemic manifestation, including stable, unstable angina and myocardial infarction.[5,14,30–36] A recent study from our laboratory has shown that in patients recovering from a myocardial infarction and who underwent an adenosine thallium-201 SPECT study an average of 5 days after the infarction, the findings on adenosine thallium SPECT were very accurate for predicting future cardiac events. In that study, coronary angiography was not as good a predictor of cardiac events.[35,36] Cerqueira et al.[37] previously demonstrated that quantification of perfusion defect size on rest thallium-201 SPECT allowed a good discrimination between patients with a low risk for subsequent cardiac events (death or recurrent infarction) identified by a defect size ≤15% of the left ventricle, and those with a high risk for events, who had a defect size involving ≥15% of the left ventricle.

Myocardial perfusion scintigraphy during pharmacologic vasodilation is a useful adjunct to the risk stratification of selected patients undergoing noncardiac operations, especially vascular surgeries.[38-40]

Transient exercise-induced perfusion defects in patients with hypertrophic cardiomyopathy identify patients who are at increased risk for subsequent death.[41]

Assessment of Myocardial Viability

It stands to reason that revascularization of myocardial scar per se would not be expected to produce any clinical or functional benefits. On the other hand, in areas of chronically hypoperfused myocardium, where the hypoperfusion led to a chronic decrease in myocardial contraction (with or without heart failure), the reestablishment of coronary flow should lead to improved perfusion and enhanced cardiac function—and hopefully to an improved prognosis. These concepts have spearheaded the quest to identify reversibly hypoperfused, hypocontractile myocardium that is still viable and hence could improve after revascularization.

Viable myocardium can be identified by perfusion scintigraphy when: (1) there is a normal tracer uptake during stress or at rest; (2) there is hypoperfusion during stress that improves with redistribution or after thallium-201 reinjection;[42-45] (3) when the rest or stress perfusion defect still contains $\geq 50\%$ of the normal tracer uptake; (4) when a rest perfusion defect redistributes over time (4 to 24 hr). Most of the accumulated experience with detection of viability by perfusion scintigraphy has used thallium-201 as a tracer. Recent evidence, however, suggests that even with ^{99m}Tc sestamibi, the presence of 50% or more tracer uptake in the defects is a good marker of viable myocardium.

Another possible marker of myocardium viability is the uptake of iodine-123 iodophenyl pentadecanoic acid (IPPA). Preliminary results on a large multicenter trial suggest that preserved uptake of IPPA in patients with myocardial dysfunction is an alternative marker of viable myocardium and improved function after coronary revascularization.[46]

Perhaps the most sophisticated technique to assess myocardial viability is positron emission tomography (PET). The presence of a mismatch between flow (determined by nitrogen-13 ammonia, rubidium-82, or oxygen-15 water) and uptake of fluorine-18 fluordeoxyglucose (18-FDG) is a strong predictor of poor prognosis with medical therapy and improved prognosis and enhanced cardiac function after revascularization.[47,48] Because of the limited availability of PET and the high costs involved, PET remains confined to relatively few medical centers around the world.

Contraindications

Myocardial perfusion imaging is contraindicated in pregnant or lactating women. The only other contraindication is in patients who recently received another nuclear imaging procedure with a long half-life tracer (e.g., a gallium scan). Otherwise, with the availability of technetium-labeled compounds, even patients as large as 500 lb may be currently imaged.

With respect to the type of stress employed, exercise performed on a treadmill or on a bicycle ergometer is the preferred stress modality. Two pharmacologic stress agents are currently approved by the FDA to be used in combination with perfusion imaging: dipyridamole and adenosine. The mechanism of these two agents is similar, i.e., interaction with the adenosine A2 receptors in the coronary arteries, leading to coronary vasodilation. Although both are effective vasodilators, adenosine has the advantage of an ultrashort half-life (<10 sec), the ability to be titrated up or down, and possibly a more complete coronary vasodilation. Both dipyridamole and adenosine are contraindicated in patients with asthma or bronchospasm, those with advanced degrees of atrioventricular block, those who have severe hypotension, or with allergy to these compounds (an extremely rare event). Adenosine also should not be given to patients using oral dipyridamole, unless the latter is discontinued for at least 24 hr. Moreover, neither dipyridamole nor adenosine should be given to patients with recent use (<24 hr) of teophylline or caffeine compounds, because these will competitively block the adenosine receptors.

Dobutamine is another agent that has been used for several years for pharmacologic stress in combination with perfusion imaging.[3,10]

Advantages and Disadvantages

Myocardial perfusion imaging is the best validated noninvasive technique for the assessment of CAD. The disadvantages of perfusion imaging are that it requires a small dose of radiation and necessitates a gamma camera. Although the tracers are not cheap, the prices have decreased in recent years due to competitive market forces. The new, sophisticated tomographic gamma cameras are expensive, but fortunately are reliable, sturdy pieces of equipment that function well for many years.

Stress echocardiography has been used in recent years for the evaluation of CAD. Although stress echocardiography (with exercise or dobutamine) is a reasonable alternative for this purpose, and has the advantages of not requiring any radioactivity and being slightly less expensive than a nuclear cardiac imaging procedure, it cannot assess disturbances in myocardial blood flow, which is the hallmark of CAD. A detailed comparison between myocardial perfusion imaging and stress 2D echocardiography has been recently reported.[49] Positron emission tomography, of course, is a superior technique for the assessment of myocardial blood flow, however, it remains a very expensive technique and is not widely available.

Although magnetic resonance imaging has been performed during dobutamine stress for the evaluation of CAD, this technique has not made it into the clinical arena as yet.

The treadmill exercise testing alone remains useful for selected patients and affords useful prognostic information, but its limited sensitivity and specificity make it less accurate in comparison to myocardial perfusion imaging for the assessment of CAD.

Future Advancement

Recent refinements in the techniques of photon attenuation–correction are expected to enhance the value of perfusion imaging, especially with respect to the clarification of artifacts caused by excessive photon attenuation.

New myocardial tracers are likely to become available in the coming years, both for the study of myocardial perfusion and myocardial metabolism with SPECT. An agent with higher myocardial extraction fraction, especially during hyperemia— where most of the available tracers exhibit a diminished extraction—and a low liver and lung uptake would be very welcome in nuclear cardiology. Myocardial SPECT with simultaneous evaluation of myocardial perfusion and ventricular function by using gated tomography with automatic image quantification may become routine in the near future. Further improvements in gamma camera technology and computer techniques will certainly continue to enhance the ultimate clinical value of perfusion imaging.

Special Considerations

The cost-effectiveness of myocardial perfusion imaging can be best demonstrated by applying it to patients with an intermediate or high pretest probability of coronary artery disease. The powerful negative predictive value of a normal myocardial perfusion scan can be used to select patients who need coronary angiography and therefore may curtail the number of unnecessary coronary angiography procedures and the number of normal coronary angiography reports. Likewise, in patients with myocardial infarction or unstable angina, myocardial perfusion imaging is more cost-effective than routine coronary angiography and therefore should be used to select patients who are at high risk for events and who should then undergo coronary angiography. Such a strategy could markedly decrease the number of patients currently undergoing coronary angiography after acute infarction or unstable angina, with substantial cost savings.

Radionuclide Angiography

Technical Considerations

Radionuclide angiography is usually done using either a blood pool, gated equilibrium technique or a first-pass technique. The blood pool technique is performed after labeling the patient's red blood cells with ^{99m}Tc and has the advantage that acquisitions can be repeated for several hours after the labeling procedure. Multiple views can be acquired at rest and then during stress. A major advantage of blood pool radionuclide angiography is that it can be done with the simplest of the gamma cameras, capable of doing only planar imaging. First-pass radionuclide angiography, on the other hand, requires specialized gamma cameras with a high-counting rate to be optimally done. Two types of specialized gamma cameras for first-pass radionuclide angiography are available: the multicrystal gamma camera, which uses ^{99m}Tc as a tracer, and the multiwire gamma camera, which uses low-energy, short-lived tracers such as tantalum-178 or iridium-191m.[50,51]

Developmental Perspectives

Both first-pass and equilibrium blood pool radionuclide angiography developed concurrently but independently two decades ago. Two excellent historical perspectives of these two techniques have been recently reported.[52,53] Both of these techniques have come a long way since their first introduction, in great part because of technological refinements in gamma camera and computer technology. Radionuclide angiography at the present time can be done with portable devices, with high degree of reproducibility and with computer quantification of ventricular function parameters.

Indications And Uses

The indications for radionuclide angiography are listed in Table 2.2. In short, radionuclide angiography is probably the most accurate and reproducible available technique to assess left and right ventricular function. The parameters that can be measured by radionuclide angiography are listed in Table 2.3. The major advantage of radionuclide angiography over other techniques that can also assess ventricular function is that it routinely uses computer quantification of systolic and diastolic ventricular function parameters, hence it is more reproducible and accurate.

The most compelling reason to perform radionuclide angiography is to assess the left ventricular ejection fraction, which has a major prognostic value in patients with heart diseases of different etiologies. Radionuclide angiography is particularly useful in the assessment of ventricular function in patients with congestive heart failure secondary to CAD, mitral or aortic valvular lesions, or dilated cardiomyopathies. In patients with chronic CAD, as well as in those recovering from a recent myocardial infarction, the left ventricular ejection fraction is one of the most important prognostic indicators.[54,55] In patients with suspected right ventricular infarction, radionuclide angiography may be the most sensitive means to detect right ventricular dysfunction.

Radionuclide angiography is often performed during exercise in patients with suspected or documented coronary artery disease. In these patients, one can often elicit deterioration of regional wall motion during exercise, as well as a fall in left ventricular ejection fraction. Such an abnormal response can be reversed by successful myocardial revascularization by coronary angioplasty[56–58] or coronary artery bypass graft surgery.[59]

Radionuclide angiography at times may be very useful in patients with low cardiac output after open heart surgeries. The response of the left ventricular ejection fraction to manipulations of the pumping flow rates in patients on a left ventricular

TABLE 2.2.   Indications for RNA

Assessment of Left and Right Ventricular Function
   In patients with documented or suspected CAD (diagnosis, prognosis)
   In patients with valvular lesions
   Postmyocardial infarction (left and right ventricles)
   In patients with CHF (including cor pulmonale and pre–lung transplant)
   To assess therapeutic intervention (PTCA, CABG, medical therapy)
   In patients with low cardiac output after open-heart surgery
   Before and during chemotherapy

Abbreviations: CABG = coronary artery bypass graft surgery; CAD = coronary artery disease; CHF = congestive heart failure; PTCA = percutaneous transluminal coronary angioplasty.

TABLE 2.3.   Radionuclide-derived Measurements

1. Left ventricular function
   a. Ejection fraction: global and regional
   b. Volumes
   c. Wall motion
   d. Regurgitant fraction
   e. Diastolic function: global and regional
2. Right ventricular function
   a. Ejection fraction
   b. Wall motion
   c. Volumes
   d. Regurgitant fraction
3. Intracardiac shunts
4. Mean pulmonary transit time
5. Pulmonary blood volume
6. Cardiac output
7. Impulse conduction and propagation
8. Pericardial effusion
9. Peripheral hemodynamics
10. Splanchnic hemodynamics

From: Iskandrian AS, Verani MS: Radionuclide angiography. In *Nuclear Cardiac Imaging: Principles and Applications.* Philadelphia, FA Davis, 1996, pp 144–218. Reproduced with permission.

assist device is useful in identifying patients who will be successfully weaned from the assist device.[60]

Contraindications

Radionuclide angiography has very few contraindications. As usual, pregnant or lactating females should not receive a radionuclide injection. Patients who recently underwent another radionuclide procedure (e.g., lung scan, gallium scan, or a cardiac perfusion scan with one of the technetium tracers) must be assessed on an individual basis for a possible cross-talk of the tracers. Patients with very irregular heart rhythms (e.g., atrial fibrillation with wide variation of R-R intervals, or frequent premature ventricular contractions) may at times post a difficult technical problem because of the inability to perform stable electrocardiographic gating.

Advantages and Disadvantages

Although prices often are considered to be more than with echocardiography, current hospital charges are nearly comparable in patients undergoing rest 2D echocardiography or radionuclide angiography.

   Echocardiography also remains a technique that is highly dependent on a good echocardiographic window. Consequently, very large patients and those with pulmonary disease often have poor images by 2D echocardiography which renders a proper evaluation of ventricular function difficult if not impossible.

Future Advancement

Relatively small, portable gamma cameras already exist and are useful to perform bedside examinations, but it is conceivable that even smaller detectors would facilitate the more widespread use of radionuclide angiography in the coronary care unit or intensive care unit.

A very significant advantage of the technetium-labeled perfusion tracers is that they can be used for first-pass radionuclide angiography during the injection of the tracer. Thus, one can obtain perfusion images as well as radionuclide angiography following one injection of a single tracer. At the present time, this requires a multicrystal gamma camera to obtain optimal count statistics, but some of the newer cameras with high count-rate capability may also prove useful for this purpose.

CONCLUSION

Nuclear cardiology has come a long way in the last two decades. The powerful diagnostic and prognostic value of myocardial perfusion imaging and radionuclide angiography has been established beyond any doubt. Yet, much remains to be done in disseminating this information and making it available with consistent proficiency and at low cost. Myocardial perfusion imaging remains the most useful noninvasive technique for the assessment of patients with CAD, because it directly assesses myocardial perfusion. Because this disease primarily affects the myocardial perfusion and only secondarily the wall motion, techniques that assess perfusion directly such as SPECT perfusion imaging are superior to techniques that assess wall motion, such as radionuclide angiography or 2D echocardiography.

With respect to ventricular function assessment, radionuclide angiography remains the most accurate, quantitative, and reproducible noninvasive technique available. Future technological advances in gamma camera technology and their computers will in all likelihood further enhance the clinical value of these techniques.

REFERENCES

1. Gould KL: Noninvasive assessment of coronary stenoses by myocardial perfusion imaging during pharmacologic coronary vasodilation: I. Physiologic basis and experimental validation. *Am J Cardiol* 41:267–278, 1978.
2. Gould KL, Westcott RJ, Albro PC, et al: Noninvasive assessment of coronary stenosis by myocardial imaging during pharmacologic coronary vasodilatation: II. Clinical methodology and feasibility. *Am J Cardiol* 41:279–287, 1978.
3. Iskandrian AS, Verani MS: *Nuclear Cardiac Imaging. Principles and Applications.* Philadelphia, FA Davis, 1996.
4. Mahmarian JJ, Verani MS: Exercise thallium-201 perfusion scintigraphy in the assessment of coronary heart disease. *Am J Cardiol* 67:2D–11D, 1991.
5. Iskandrian AS, Verani MS: Risk assessment. In Iskandrian AS, Verani MS: *Nuclear Cardiac Imaging. Principles and Applications*. Philadelphia, FA Davis, 1996, p 242.

6. Rozanski A, Diamond GA, Berman D, et al: The declining specificity of exercise radionu-clide ventriculography. *N Engl J Med* 309:518–522, 1983.

7. Nallamothu N, Pancholy SB, Lee KR, et al: Impact of exercise single-photon emission computed tomographic thallium imaging on patient management and outcome. *J Nucl Cardiol* 2:334–338, 1995.

8. Dakik HA, Kimball K, Vaduganathan P, et al: The impact of clinical history, exercise parameters and myocardial perfusion tomographic variables on the selection of patients for coronary angiography (abstract). *Circulation* 92:I522, 1995.

9. Zaret BL, Beller GA: *Nuclear Cardiology. State of the Art and Future Directions.* St Louis, Mosby, 1992.

10. Nuclear cardiology: state of the art. *Cardiol Clin* 12:169–391, 1994, Verani MS, guest editor. Philadelphia, WB Saunders, 1994.

11. Gerson MC: *Cardiac Nuclear Medicine.* New York, McGraw-Hill, 1991.

12. Iskandrian AS, Van der Wall EE: Myocardial viability. Detection and clinical relevance. Dordrecht, Kluwer Academic Publishers, 1994.

13. DePuey EG, Berman DS, Garcia EV: *Cardiac SPECT Imaging.* New York, Raven Press, 1995.

14. Beller GA: *Clinical Nuclear Cardiology.* Philadelphia, WB Saunders, 1995.

15. Bilodeau L, Theroux P, Gregoire J, et al: Technetium-99m-sestamibi tomography in patients with spontaneous chest pain: correlations with clinical, electrocardiographic and angiographic findings. *J Am Coll Cardiol* 18:1684–1691, 1991.

16. Varetto T, Cantalupi D, Altieri A, et al: Emergency room technetium-99m sestamibi imaging to rule out acute myocardial ischemic events in patients with nondiagnostic elec-trocardiograms. *J Am Coll Cardiol* 22:1804–1808, 1993.

17. Fuller CM, Raizner AE, Chahine RA, et al: Exercise-induced coronary arterial spasm: angiographic demonstration, documentation of ischemia by myocardial scintigraphy and results of pharmacologic intervention. *Am J Cardiol* 46:500–506, 1980.

18. Gallik DM, Mahmarian JJ, Verani MS: Therapeutic significance of exercise-induced ST-segment elevation in patients without previous myocardial infarction. *Am J Cardiol* 72:1–7, 1993.

19. Miller DD, Verani MS: Current status of myocardial perfusion imaging following percu-taneous transluminal coronary angioplasty. *J Am Coll Cardiol* 24:260–266, 1994.

20. Jain A, Mahmarian JJ, Borges-Neto S, et al: Clinical significance of perfusion defects by thallium-201 single photon emission tomography following oral dipyridamole early after coronary angioplasty. *J Am Coll Cardiol* 11:970–976, 1988.

21. Lakkis NM, Mahmarian JJ, Verani MS: Exercise thallium-201 single photon emission computed tomography for evaluation of coronary artery bypass graft patency. *Am J Car-diol* 76:107–111, 1995.

22. Zacca NM, Verani MS, Chahine RA, et al: Effect of nifedipine on exercise-induced left ventricular dysfunction and myocardial hypoperfusion in stable angina. *Am J Cardiol* 50:689–695, 1982.

23. Mahmarian JJ, Moyé LA, Verani MS, et al: High reproducibility of myocardial perfusion defects in patients undergoing serial exercise thallium-201 tomography. *Am J Cardiol* 75:1116–1119, 1995.

24. Verani MS, Jeroudi MO, Mahmarian JJ, et al: Quantification of myocardial infarction during coronary occlusion and myocardial salvage after reperfusion using cardiac imag-ing with technetium-99m hexakis 2-methoxyisobutyl isonitrile. *J Am Coll Cardiol* 12:1573–1581, 1988.

25. Wackers FJT, Gibbons RJ, Verani MS, et al: Serial quantitative planar technetium-99m-isonitrile imaging in acute myocardial infarction: efficacy for noninvasive assessment of thrombolytic therapy. *J Am Coll Cardiol* 14:861–873, 1989.

26. Gibbons RJ, Verani MS, Behrenbeck T, et al: Feasibility of tomographic technetium-99m-hexakis-2-methoxy-2-methylpropyl-isonitrile imaging for the assessment of myocardial area at risk and the effect of acute treatment in myocardial infarction. *Circulation* 80:1277–1286, 1989.

27. Gibbons RJ, Holmes DR, Reeder GS, et al: Immediate angioplasty compared with the administration of a thrombolytic agent followed by conservative treatment for myocardial infarction. *N Engl J Med* 328:685–691, 1993.

28. Mahmarian JJ, Pratt CM, Borges-Neto S, et al: Quantification of infarct size by ^{201}Tl single-photon emission computed tomography during acute myocardial infarction in humans: comparison with enzymatic estimates. *Circulation* 78:831–839, 1988.

29. Tamaki S, Nakajima H, Murakami T, et al: Estimation of infarct size by myocardial emission computed tomography with thallium-201 and its relation to creatine kinase-MB release after a myocardial infarction in man. *Circulation* 66:994–1001, 1982.

30. Heller GV, Brown KA: Prognosis of acute and chronic coronary artery disease by myocardial perfusion imaging. *Cardiol Clin* 12:271–288, 1994.

31. Brown KA: Prognostic value of thallium-201 myocardial perfusion imaging. A diagnostic tool comes of age. *Circulation* 83:363–381, 1991.

32. Iskandrian AS, Chae SC, Heo J, et al: Independent and incremental prognostic value of exercise thallium tomographic imaging in coronary artery disease. *J Am Coll Cardiol* 22:665–670, 1993.

33. Gibson RS, Watson DD, Craddock GB, et al: Prediction of cardiac events after uncomplicated myocardial infarction: a prospective study comparing predischarge exercise thallium-201 scintigraphy and coronary angiography. *Circulation* 68:321–336, 1983.

34. Leppo JA, O'Brien J, Rothendler JA, et al: Dipyridamole thallium-201 scintigraphy in the prediction of future cardiac events after acute myocardial infarction. *N Engl J Med* 310:1014–1018, 1984.

35. Mahmarian JJ, Pratt CM, Nishimura S, et al: Quantitative adenosine thallium-201 single-photon emission computed tomography for the early assessment of patients surviving acute myocardial infarction. *Circulation* 87:1197–1210, 1993.

36. Mahmarian JJ, Mahmarian AC, Marks GF, et al: Role of adenosine thallium-201 tomography for defining long-term risk in patients after acute myocardial infarction. *J Am Coll Cardiol* 25:1333–1340, 1995.

37. Cerqueira MD, Maynard C, Ritchie JL, et al: Long-term survival in 618 patients from the Western Washington Streptokinase in Myocardial Infarction trials. *J Am Coll Cardiol* 20:1452–1459, 1992.

38. Leppo J, Plaja J, Gionet M, et al: Noninvasive evaluation of cardiac risk before elective vascular surgery. *J Am Coll Cardiol* 9:269–276, 1987.

39. Hendel RC, Whitfield SS, Villegas BJ, et al: Prediction of late cardiac events by dipyridamole thallium imaging in patients undergoing elective vascular surgery. *Am J Cardiol* 70:1243–1249, 1992.

40. Koutelou MG, Asimacopoulos PJ, Mahmarian JJ, et al: Preoperative risk stratification by adenosine thallium-201 single-photon emission computed tomography in patients undergoing vascular surgery. *J Nucl Cardiol* 2:389–394, 1995.

41. Dilsizian V, Bonow RO, Epstein SE, et al: Myocardial ischemia detected by thallium

scintigraphy is frequently related to cardiac arrest and syncope in young patients with hypertrophic cardiomyopathy. *J Am Coll Cardiol* 22:796–804, 1993.

42. Iskandrian AS, Verani SM: Myocardial viability. In Iskandrian AS, Verani MS: *Nuclear Cardiac Imaging: Principles and Applications.* Philadelphia, FA Davis, 1996, p 305.

43. Dilsizian V, Rocco TP, Freedman NMT, et al: Enhanced detection of ischemic but viable myocardium by the reinjection of thallium after stress-redistribution imaging. *N Engl J Med* 323:141–146, 1990.

44. Dilsizian V, Bonow RO: Current diagnostic techniques of assessing myocardial viability in patients with hibernating and stunned myocardium. *Circulation* 87:1–20, 1993.

45. Dilsizian V, Arrighi JA, Diodati JG, et al: Myocardial viability in patients with chronic coronary artery disease. Comparison of Tc-99m sestamibi with thallium reinjection and F-18-fluorodeoxyglucose. *Circulation* 89:578–587, 1994.

46. Verani MS, Taillefer R, Mahmarian JJ, et al: I-123 Iodophenylpentadecanoic acid (IPPA) metabolic imaging predicts improvement of global left ventricular function after coronary revascularization (abstract). *J Am Coll Cardiol* 1996; 27 (suppl) 300A.

47. Schelbert HR: Blood flow metabolism by PET. *Cardiol Clin* 12:303–317, 1994.

48. Di Carli MF, Davidson M, Little R, et al: Value of metabolic imaging with positron emission tomography for evaluating prognosis in patients with coronary artery disease and left ventricular dysfunction. *Am J Cardiol* 73:527–533, 1994.

49. Verani MS: Myocardial perfusion imaging versus 2D echocardiography: comparative value in the diagnosis of coronary artery disease. *J Nucl Cardiol* 1:399–414, 1994.

50. Lacy JL, Verani MS, Ball ME, et al: First-pass radionuclide angiography using a multi-wire gamma camera and tantalum-178. *J Nucl Med* 29:293–301, 1988.

51. Verani MS, Lacy JL, Guidry GW, et al: Quantification of left ventricular performance during transient coronary occlusion at various anatomic sites in humans: a study using tantalum-178 and a multiwire gamma camera. *J Am Coll Cardiol* 19:297–306, 1992.

52. Borer JS, Supino P, Wencker D, et al: Assessment of coronary artery disease by radionuclide cineangiography. History, current applications, and new directions. *Cardiol Clin* 12:333–357, 1994.

53. Port SC: Recent advances in first-pass radionuclide angiography. *Cardiol Clin* 12:359–372, 1994.

54. CASS Principal Investigators and their associates: Coronary artery surgery study (CASS): a randomized trial of coronary artery bypass surgery: survival data. *Circulation* 68:939–950, 1983.

55. Multicenter Postinfarction Research Group: Risk stratification and survival after myocardial infarction. *N Engl J Med* 309:331–336, 1983.

56. De Puey EG, Leatherman LL, Chermiles J, et al: Restenosis after transluminal coronary angioplasty detected with exercise-gated radionuclide angiography. *J Am Coll Cardiol* 4:1103–1113, 1984.

57. Lewis JF, Verani MS, Poliner LR, et al: Effects of transluminal coronary angioplasty on left ventricular systolic and diastolic function at rest and during exercise. *Am Heart J* 109:792–798, 1985.

58. Kent KM, Bonow RO, Rosing DR, et al: Improved myocardial function during exercise after successful percutaneous transluminal coronary angioplasty. *N Engl J Med* 306:441–446, 1982.

59. Kent KM, Borer JS, Green MV, et al: Effects of coronary artery bypass on global and regional left ventricular function during exercise. *N Engl J Med* 298:1434–1439, 1978.

60. Verani MS, Sekela ME, Mahmarian JJ, et al: Left ventricular function in patients with centrifugal left ventricular assist device. *ASAIO Trans* 35:544–547, 1989.

— 3 —

Positron Emission Tomography

A. Iain McGhie, M.D.

DESCRIPTION OF THE TECHNIQUE

Positrons are emitted, along with an electron neutrino, from unstable nuclei, typically elements with a low atomic number. Positrons have the same mass as electrons but have a positive charge. The positrons travel a short distances (1–3 mm) through tissue before colliding with an electron. When this occurs, the mass and kinetic energy of the positron and the electron are converted into electromagnetic γ-radiation. This is termed an annihilation event. The electromagnetic γ-radiation consists of two high-energy (511 keV) photons emitted at approximately 180° to each other. When such a pair of photons are detected simultaneously or almost simultaneously (5–20 nanoseconds) by a pair of scintillation detectors, connected by coincidence electrical circuitry, an annihilation event is recorded (Figure 3.1). Any other scintillation events are not registered. By this means, only events occurring within the field of view of the detectors are detected with all others being discarded. This form of electronic collimation using coincidence counting in positron emission tomography (PET) is more sensitive than is used with conventional radionuclide imaging where lead collimators are used. Numerous coincidence vents are recorded by multiple (1,000–1,500) opposing scintillation detectors which are usually arranged in multiple (3–8) circular arrays. To improve data collection, the banks of detectors move to compensate for the gaps between the detectors. The coincidence data are stored and processed in a computer. Using filtered backprojection, these one-dimensional data are reconstructed into two-dimensional tomographic images. The images are corrected for attenuation which still occurs despite the relatively high energy of the

51

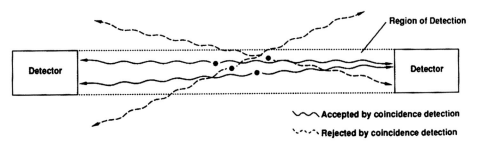

Figure 3.1. Coincidence detection. Following an annihilation reaction a pair of 511 keV photons leave at 180° from each other. They are detected by scintillation detectors connected by coincidence circuitry. From Schelbert HR: Principles of Positron Emission Tomography. In Marcus, Schelbert, Skorton (eds). *Cardiac Imaging*, WB Saunders, 1991, p 1153.

511 keV photons. Attenuation correction is performed by acquiring a transmission scan prior to the emission scan using a radioactive source, either a ring or rod, that is external to the patient.

TECHNICAL CONSIDERATIONS

Radioisotopes

Several positron-emitting radioisotopes are used in PET imaging. Typically, these radioisotopes have a short physical half-life (rubidium-82, $t_{1/2}$ = 76 sec; oxygen-15, $t_{1/2}$ = 2.1 min; carbon-11, $t_{1/2}$ = 20.4 min; nitrogen-13, $t_{1/2}$ = 10 min; fluorine-18, $t_{1/2}$ 110 min). The short half-life minimizes the radiation burden to the patient and allows sequential studies to be performed over a short period of time. In addition, O-15, C-11, and N-13 can be incorporated into metabolic substrates used by the heart. As these radioisotopes are chemically indistinct from their nonradioactive counterparts, radiolabeled substrates behave in an identical physiologic manner allowing evaluation of the metabolic processes in the myocardium using PET. However, synthesis of these radiolabeled substrates requires sophisticated technical skills and technologies and the short half-life of many of these radioisotopes mandates an on-site cyclotron which limits the availability of this technique. However, there are positron-emitting radioisotopes that are generator-produced. These include rubidium-82 and copper-62 pyruvaldehyde bis thiosemicarbazone. Rb-82 is produced from its parent compound strontium-82 which has a half-life of 25 days and is available commercially. More recently, there has been interest in PTSM copper (II) (Cu-PTSM) ($t_{1/2}$ = 9.7 min) which is also generator-produced and has been used successfully in evaluating myocardial perfusion.[1] Availability of generator-produced positron-emitting isotopes makes it possible for institutions to perform positron tomography without the requirement for costly on-site cyclotrons.

INDICATIONS AND USES

The indications and uses of positron emission tomography are shown in Table 3.1.

TABLE 3.1. Indications and Uses of Positron Emission Tomography (PET)

1. Evaluation of myocardial perfusion
   a. Detection of coronary artery disease
   b. Evaluation of patients with known or suspected coronary artery disease (progression and regression).
   c. Quantitation of myocardial blood flow
2. Evaluation of myocardial metabolism
3. Evaluation of myocardial viability

Evaluation of Myocardial Perfusion

Physiologic Basis of Stress PET Myocardial Perfusion Imaging

Since the initial distribution of myocardial perfusion tracers is primarily dependent on coronary flow, knowledge of the physiology of coronary circulation is key to understanding the basic principles of myocardial perfusion imaging. Normally, under resting basal conditions, the coronary vascular system is a low-flow, high-resistance system. This is transformed into a high-flow, low-resistance system with exercise or coronary vasodilators. At rest, coronary flow is normal even in the presence of a narrowing ≤85% diameter stenosis.[2] However, the ability of coronary flow to increase with stress begins to decrease at 40% to 50% diameter stenosis. Stress can be performed using either dynamic exercise or pharmacologic stress. Pharmacologic stress is provided using either a vasodilator, i.e., dipyridamole or adenosine, or a sympathomimetic agent, e.g., dobutamine. During stress, a normal coronary artery increases flow 2–2.5 fold with dynamic exercise and 3–4 fold with coronary vasodilators.[3-7] The increase in coronary flow during stress can be expressed as coronary flow reserve (stress/rest coronary flow). However, in the presence of a coronary stenosis, the ability of flow to increase with stress is attenuated, i.e., coronary flow reserve is reduced. In an artery with a significant stenosis, the resistance vessels are already dilated under basal conditions and are unable to dilate to the same extent as resistance vessels in normal arteries. Therefore, despite an increase in flow proximally, there is an increase in the pressure gradient across the stenosis resulting in a drop in pressure and flow distal to the stenosis. This results in a heterogeneous distribution of blood flow during stress, with a greater increase in myocardial perfusion in areas subtended by normal coronary arteries relative to the myocardium supplied by stenotic arteries. Therefore, the distribution of a myocardial perfusion agent administered during stress, e.g., Rb-82 or N-13 ammonia, will also be heterogeneous in the presence of a hemodynamically significant coronary stenosis. This heterogeneity is reflected in the tomographic images as an area of reduced uptake of the tracer.

In certain circumstances, coronary flow distal to the stenosis may actually decrease during stress, i.e., myocardial steal, resulting in subendocardial ischemia. This can occur in two circumstances: (1) In the presence of one or more diseased vessels with collaterals between their respective distal beds. During stress, if an unequal fall in pressure occurs between these distal perfusion beds, blood is shunted away from the distal bed with the higher perfusion pressure to the one with the lower perfusion pressure. This is referred to as *horizontal steal*. (2) In the presence of a single severe coronary stenosis, the coronary pressure distal to the stenosis may decrease enough during stress that it is insufficient to perfuse the endocardium resulting in ischemia despite an increase in total flow in the proximal epicardial artery. This is sometimes referred to as *vertical steal*.

Myocardial perfusion can be evaluated in patients using either diffusible tracers, e.g., O-15-labeled water or by using extractable tracers, e.g., Rb-82, N-13 ammonia, Cu-PTSM. There are experimental data which show a very close correlation between the myocardial distribution of microspheres and O-15-labeled water over a wide variation in coronary flows.[8,9] Because O-15-labeled water labels both the cardiac blood pool as well as the myocardium, a means of correction is required. This is usually performed using inhaled O-15-labeled carbon monoxide which rapidly labels red blood cells which is subtracted from the O-15-labeled water study. Although this technique has been used successfully to evaluate myocardial perfusion under a variety of clinical scenarios, it is generally reserved only for use as a research tool. Because of the increased complexity of this technique, myocardial perfusion is more commonly assessed using the extractable tracers, e.g., Rb-82, N-13 ammonia. This group of tracers has been extensively used in the assessment of myocardial perfusion. It is assumed that these tracers are distributed to and retained by the myocardium in relation to coronary blood flow. This assumption is not entirely valid as extraction of N-13 ammonia is inversely and nonlinearly related to coronary flow and plateaus at flows greater than 2.5 ml/gm/min to 3.0 mg/gm/ml.[10] Despite this, N-13 ammonia has a high first-pass extraction with rapid blood pool clearance and a relatively long residence in the myocardium and generally provides very good quality images. Typically, 10–15 mCi of N-13 ammonia is injected intravenously; after a 4-min delay to allow for clearance of blood pool activity, data for 10–15 min is acquired. Forty minutes after injection of the first dose of N-13 ammonia, dipyridamole is infused in a dose 0.142 mg/kg/min over 4 min. Two minutes later, handgrip is begun for 4 min, with the stress injection of N-13 ammonia (10–15 mCi) being injected 2 min into the handgrip.

Rubidium-82 uptake is also nonlinearly related to flow with an underestimation at coronary flow rates > 2.5 mg/gm/min to 3.0 mg/gm/min.[11] It has the advantage of being generator-produced and a short $t_{1/2}$ of 75 sec which allows for rapid imaging without need of an on-site cyclotron. Generally, 30–50 mCi is injected in 10 ml volume over 20–30 sec with a fresh generator; later towards the end of the generator life (6 wk), 30–40 ml is required to deliver a similar dose of Rb-82. Data is acquired for 5 to 8 min with the second stress dose being administered 10 min later as described for N-13 ammonia. Rb-82 has been very successfully used in a number of clinical studies for the assessment of myocardial perfusion and a generator (CardioGen-82, Squibb Diagnostics) has been commercially available for several years.

Detection of Coronary Artery Disease

The superior spatial resolution and the ability to perform attenuation correction made PET imaging one of the most accurate noninvasive techniques currently available for the detection of coronary heart disease. Several published studies report a sensitivity of between 82–98% and a specificity of 82–100%, with a mean sensitivity and specificity of 91% and 90%, respectively.[12–17]

Evaluation of Patients with Known or Suspected Coronary Artery Disease

Although myocardial perfusion imaging is widely used in the diagnosis of coronary artery disease, it is perhaps in the functional assessment of patients with already documented coronary disease that these techniques are most useful. There already exists a large body of literature attesting to the utility of conventional SPECT imaging in determining prognosis in patients with coronary artery disease.[18] Due to the more limited availability of PET, such data does not exist. However, there is no reason to believe that PET does not provide at least equivalent data.

Assessment of Regression of Coronary Stenoses

More recently, there has been much interest in the use of aggressive lipid-lowering therapies to arrest and regress coronary artery disease with several large trials showing angiographic regression of coronary disease associated with reduction in clinical events.[19] Gould and associates have utilized serial PET to follow patients undergoing aggressive lipid-lowering therapy.[20,21] They have shown improvement in the extent and the severity of myocardial perfusion defects with lipid lowering detected by PET. In addition, they observed that these improvements in myocardial perfusion often occur before any improvements in the coronary angiogram become apparent. This raises the interesting possibility that the improvements in myocardial perfusion reflect improved endothelial function that occurs with cholesterol reduction. Grambow and associates have shown, using cold-pressor testing and PET, evidence of endothelial dysfunction in patients with angiographically mild coronary artery disease.[22] There is also evidence of impaired coronary flow reserve in asymptomatic individuals without clinically apparent CAD but who have high risk factor profiles for developing CAD.[23]

Quantitation of Myocardial Blood Flow

Unlike SPECT imaging, PET can also be used to quantitate noninvasively absolute myocardial blood flow in terms of mg/gm/min. Technically, this is more complex and more demanding both in terms of data acquisition and also data processing. However, several approaches have been successful in providing reproducible determinations of absolute myocardial blood flow using both O-15 labeled water and N-13 ammonia.[24–27] Although these techniques have important research applications, whether this additional information over and above the qualitative assessments of myocardial blood flow will be clinically useful is uncertain at this time. However, it may provide clinicians with a means of more accurately determining the physiologic significance of coronary artery disease that is detected or undetected by the coronary angiogram.[28]

Evaluation of Myocardial Metabolism

As discussed earlier, labeling substrates with positron-emitting isotopes allows evaluation of myocardial metabolism with positron tomography. The labeled compounds that have been most widely used in the field of myocardial metabolism have been fluorine-18 fluorodeoxyglucose, carbon-11-labeled palmitate, and carbon-11-labeled acetate.

Fluorine-18 Fluorodeoxyglucose

Under fasting conditions, fatty acids are the main energy source of normal myocardium. In the presence of ischemia, the myocardium increases its utilization of glucose as a source of high-energy phosphates. This enhanced utilization of glucose as an energy source by ischemic myocardium can be estimated with PET using fluorine-18 fluorodeoxyglucose (FDG). This radiolabeled intermediary undergoes phosphorylation by the hexokinase reaction, but it is not metabolized any further in the glycolytic pathway. Therefore, phosphorylated FDG is in essence trapped in the cytosol and accumulates in proportion to exogenous metabolism of glucose.[29,30]

Carbon-11-Labeled Palmitate

Fatty acids are the preferred substrate of the myocardium under fasting conditions accounting for approximately 90% of oxygen consumed under aerobic conditions. Carbon-11-labeled palmitate has been used extensively in the evaluation of myocardial metabolism.[31–35] Uptake is primarily dependent on blood flow, however, inferences about β-oxidation can be made by studying the subsequent washout of the radiolabeled fatty acids from the myocardium. Clearance from myocardium is biexponential, with an early fast and a slower second component. The early phase is a reflection of β-oxidation of the fatty acids, while the slower clearance results from incorporation of the fatty acids into the endogenous lipid pool. Myocardial ischemia reduces the early myocardial clearance of fatty acids because of decreased β-oxidation and increases in the proportion of fatty acid incorporated into the lipid pool.[36,37]

Carbon-11-Labeled Acetate

This radiolabeled intermediary of oxidative phosphorylation has also been used to study myocardial metabolism.[38–43] Myocardium avidly extracts acetate and is activated to acetyl-CoA in the cytosol and oxidized in mitochondria via the tricarboxylic acid cycle which is the final common pathway of oxidative metabolism. Regional time activity curves show biexponential clearance which is independent of blood flow. The rapid, early phase reflects oxidative phosphorylation and a slower, late clearance represents incorporation into the amino acid and lipid pool. Rate constants obtained from the rapid clearance of C-11 acetate are closely related to the rate of myocardial oxygen consumption over a wide range of physiologic values. In the presence of myocardial ischemia, uptake is reduced in proportion to flow and clearance is reduced in proportion to oxidative metabolism.[38–44]

Assessment of Myocardial Viability

One of the most significant contributions PET has made to clinical cardiology has been in the area of myocardial viability. Different techniques using PET have been developed to evaluate myocardial viability. These can be divided into those utilizing metabolic imaging using either F-18 FDG, C-11 acetate, or C-11 palmitate and more recently by estimating the water-perfusable tissue index (PTI).

F-18 Fluorodeoxyglucose

Mismatch of metabolism and perfusion, i.e., areas of myocardium with metabolic activity in areas but with severely reduced perfusion, has been used as a marker of hibernating myocardium. This can be identified using PET by finding normal or increased myocardial uptake of F-18 FDG in the presence of reduced uptake of a marker of myocardial perfusion, i.e., N-13 ammonia, O-15 water, or Rb-82. Assessment of myocardial viability using F-18 FDG and PET varies between institutions. Typically, patients receive 50 gm of glucose solution to change the main source of myocardial substrate utilization from fatty acids to glucose. This is followed by injection of 15–20 mCi of N-13 ammonia and resting myocardial perfusion images are acquired 5–10 min later. Patients are then injected with 10 mCi of F-18 FDG and imaged approximately 45 min later for approximately 30 min. Reconstructed tomograms and polar maps of myocardial perfusion and metabolic activity are then compared.

Myocardial blood flow–metabolism mismatch was first demonstrated by Marshall et al. in patients with prior myocardial infarction[45] (Figure 3.2). Two subsequent studies demonstrated this technique to be of value in predicting the functional outcome of revascularization in patients undergoing coronary artery surgery; the positive and negative predictive accuracies were 78%–81% and 78%–92%, respectively.[46,47] A more recent study has confirmed the high negative predictive accuracy of this technique but found that functional recovery following revascularization in myocardium with metabolism–perfusion mismatch was more variable.[48] The value of FDG in determining myocardial viability in patients following recent myocardial infarction is less certain.[48–50] These studies demonstrate that myocardium with severely reduced perfusion and a matched absence of metabolic activity is strongly predictive of lack of functional recovery either with time or following revascularization. However, the positive predictive value of finding myocardial perfusion–metabolism mismatch is much lower. For example, Schwaiger et al. found that functional recovery occurred in only 50% of segments with severely reduced perfusion and enhanced FDG uptake.[49] Despite these possible limitations following recent myocardial infarction, several retrospective studies have shown that identification of myocardial blood flow–metabolism in patients with coronary artery disease has important prognostic and therapeutic implications.[51–53] These studies have shown that patients with impaired left ventricular function and evidence of flow–metabolism mismatch have a poorer prognosis, with a higher incidence of myocardial infarction and sudden cardiac death than patients without areas of flow–metabolism mismatch. In addition, two of these studies showed that patients with a flow–metabolism mismatch who underwent revascularization had a substantially lower incidence of future cardiac events and cardiac death than those who were treated medically.

Carbon-11-Labeled Palmitate

Sobel's group has published extensively on the myocardial kinetics of C-11 palmitate kinetics and its role in determining myocardial viability in both experimental models and in humans.[33–35] However, interpreting myocardial kinetics of radiolabeled fatty acids is complex due to several compounding variables. These include blood flow, competition with alternate substrates, back-diffusion of unmetabolized

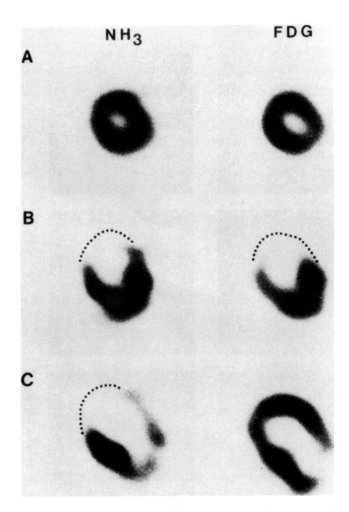

Figure 3.2. PET tomograms showing different patterns of myocardial perfusion and metabolism. The left-hand images are N-13 ammonia (NH_3) tomograms (myocardial perfusion); right-hand images are F-18 FDG tomograms (myocardial metabolism). The top row (A) shows normal myocardial perfusion and metabolism; middle row (B) shows images from a patient with an anterior-wall myocardial infarction with a severe, matched reduction in both perfusion and function consistent with nonviable myocardium; bottom row (C) shows a large anterior and septal perfusion abnormality but with enhanced FDG uptake. This myocardial perfusion–metabolism is consistent with viable myocardium. From Schelbert HR, Current status and prospects for new radionuclides and radiopharmaceuticals for cardiovascular nuclear medicine. Seminars in Nuclear Medicine. 17(2):145–181, 1987.

tracer into the vascular space, availability of other intermediate compounds, and the activity of key enzymes.[54,55] These problems along with limited availability and lack of evidence demonstrating superiority over other readily available radiotracers have prevented the widespread use of C-11 palmitate.

Carbon-11-Labeled Acetate

Experimental studies have shown that oxidative metabolism is critical for myocardial viability. Oxidative metabolism is depressed following infarction, both in infarcted

58

and adjacent segments, and is observed even after restoration of myocardial blood flow has occurred.[41,56,57] Buxton et al. in their study of reperfused canine myocardium found that oxidative metabolism and regional ventricular function demonstrated a parallel recovery with time.[58] Similarly, Groper et al. also found that oxidative metabolism was a predictor of functional recovery in patients following acute myocardial infarction and also in patients with chronic coronary artery disease and that this technique was a more reliable predictor than FDG.[48,59] However, other workers have reported conflicting findings following recent myocardial infarction and observed oxidative metabolism, as assessed by C-11 acetate, was not predictive of functional recovery in this setting.[60]

Water-Perfusable Tissue Index (PTI)

This has been proposed as an alternate means for evaluating myocardial viability using PET.[61] The paradigm for this methodology is that viable myocardium exchanges water rapidly while necrotic myocardium does not. The PTI is calculated from the transmission data and emission data from blood volume (O-15 carbon monoxide labeled red cells) and myocardial blood flow (O-15 water) studies. For any particular region of interest, the PTI is expressed as the ratio of the O-15 water-perfusable fraction to total anatomic tissue fraction. Using this technique, a PTI of ≥0.70 was predictive of functional recovery following acute myocardial infarction treated with thrombolysis. In patients with previous myocardial infarction, segments with perfusion–metabolism mismatch by N-13 ammonia–FDG imaging had higher PTI than segments considered to be nonviable because of matched defects.

Evaluation of Cardiac Sympathetic Nervous System

Humoral and Receptor Imaging

The radiolabeled analog of norepinephrine, carbon-11-labeled hydroxyephedrine, allows the study of cardiac pathophysiology of the sympathetic nervous system in patients with cardiac disease.[62] Techniques have been developed that allow the visualization of both sympathetic innervation and function using the dopamine agonist, F-18 fluorodopamine which is metabolized to 6-fluoronorepinephrine in sympathetically innervated tissues.[63] This gives the potential to evaluate neuronal uptake, vesicular translocation and β-hydroxylation, all important steps in norepinephrine synthesis. With further refinement and development, it may be possible to noninvasively evaluate both presynaptic β-receptor function using norepinephrine analogs, and postsynaptic sympathetic function using receptor imaging agents.[64,65] Several ligands to other receptors, e.g., muscarinic, serotonin, benzodiazepine, and α_1-adrenergic,[66–69] all of which may play important roles in the pathogenesis and pathophysiology of cardiovascular disease, are becoming available. However, to successfully evaluate receptors using imaging techniques requires demanding scientific methodology and mathematic modeling and at present is one of the main factors limiting the more widespread application of these techniques.

ADVANTAGES AND DISADVANTAGES

Comparison of PET with SPECT Imaging

PET offers several advantages over conventional SPECT imaging with thallium-201 and ^{99m}Tc sestamibi in the detection of coronary artery disease. The inherent superior sensitivity of PET technology results in images of higher spatial resolution. The spatial resolution of typical PET images are 6–10 mm compared to 10–15 mm in conventional SPECT images. The Achilles' heel of SPECT myocardial perfusion imaging is attenuation artifacts, particularly the inferior wall and also attenuation of the anterior wall by breast tissues in females. This is the main cause for false-positive studies. It is the ability in PET to perform attenuation correction that is the major advantage that PET has over SPECT imaging. The more homogenous representation of myocardial perfusion which results from attenuation correction translates into a significantly lower false-positive rate, i.e., higher specificity. Attenuation correction using simultaneous transmission imaging is being developed for multidetector SPECT imaging systems and initial results are encouraging.[70] These are not optimal yet; however, with further development, this may narrow the gap between PET and SPECT imaging technologies. However, currently PET images are generally of higher quality with superior spatial resolution and largely attenuation artifact free when compared to conventional SPECT images. These factors are responsible for the high sensitivity and specificity found with PET imaging. Three comparative trials have observed that PET has a superior diagnostic accuracy compared with T1-201 SPECT imaging.[14,16,17] However, the results of these studies have to be interpreted with some caution as the total number of patients studied were small and may have contained selection biases; larger prospective studies are required before a definitive decision can be made.

The main disadvantages of the PET technology are its limited availability and the significantly higher capital expenditure, running, and maintenance costs. In the current climate of containment of health care costs, the future of clinical cardiac PET imaging will depend on being able to demonstrate convincing evidence of superior diagnostic accuracy and cost-effectiveness. A recent study compared the cost-effectiveness of different strategies for the detection of coronary artery disease using previously published data on sensitivities and specificities of the different diagnostic techniques.[71] The authors estimated that in patients with a pretest likelihood of coronary artery disease of <70%, PET would outperform exercise ECG testing, thallium-201 SPECT, and angiography. Whether with wider application of PET in larger nonselected patient populations this analysis would still hold true remains unanswered.

Conclusion

Positron emission tomography is an extremely powerful technique with many applications in cardiovascular medicine. It has proven to be and continues to play a very important role as a unique research tool that has made many important contributions to understanding of the pathophysiology of many cardiovascular disorders.

PET has also a proven utility in clinical cardiologic practice, particularly in the realms of the assessment of myocardial viability and the detection and evaluation of coronary artery disease.

REFERENCES

1. Shelton ME, Green MA, Mathias CJ, et al: Assessment of regional myocardial and renal blood flow with copper-PTSM and positron emission tomography. *Circulation* 82: 990–997, 1990.

2. Gould KL, Lipscomb K, Hamilton GW: Physiologic basis for assessing critical coronary stenosis: instantaneous flow response and regional distribution during coronary hyperemia as measures of coronary flow reserve. *Am J Cardiol* 33:87–94, 1974.

3. Holmberg S, Serzysko W, Varnauskas E: Coronary circulation during heavy exercise in control subjects and patients with coronary heart disease. *Acta Med Scand* 190: 465–480, 1971.

4. Heiss HW, Barmeyer J, Wink K, et al: Studies on the regulation of myocardial bloodflow in man: training effects on bloodflow and metabolism of the healthy heart at rest and during standardized heavy exercise. *Basic Res Cardiol* 71:658–675, 1976.

5. Ferguson RJ, Cote P, Gauthier P, et al: Changes in exercise coronary sinus blood flow with training in patients with angina pectoris. *Circulation* 58:41–47, 1978.

6. Wilson RF, Laughlin DE, Ackell PH, et al: Transluminal, subselective measurement of coronary artery blood flow velocity and vasodilator reserve in man. *Circulation* 72:82–92, 1985.

7. Rossen JD, Simonetti I, Marcus ML, et al: Coronary dilation with standard dose dipyridamole and dipyridamole combined with handgrip. *Circulation* 79:566–572, 1989.

8. Bergmann SR, Fox KAA, Rand AL, et al: Quantification of regional myocardial flow in vivo with Hs15O. *Circulation* 70:724, 1984.

9. Knabb RM, Fox KAA, Sobel BE, et al: Characterization of the functional significance of subcritical coronary stenoses with $H_2^{15}O$ and positron emission tomography. *Circulation* 71:1271, 1985.

10. Schelbert HR, Phelps ME, Huang SC, et al: N-13 ammonia as an indicator of myocardial blood flow. *Circulation* 63:1259, 1981.

11. Goldstein RA, Mullani NA, Marani SK, et al: Myocardial perfusion with rubidium-82: II Effects of metabolic and pharmacologic interventions. *J Nucl Med* 24:907–915, 1983.

12. Shelbert HR, Wisenberg G, Phelps ME, et al: Non-invasive assessment of coronary artery stenoses by myocardial perfusion imaging during pharmacologic coronary vasodilation: VI. Detection of coronary artery disease in human beings with intravenous N-13 ammonia and positron emission tomography. *Am J Cardiol* 49:1197–1201, 1982.

13. McCord ME, Bacharach SL, Bonow RO, et al: Misalignment between PET transmission and emission scans: its effect on myocardial imaging. *J Nucl Med* 33:1209–1213, 1992.

14. Tamaki N, Yonekura Y, Senda M, et al: Value and limitation of stress 201-Tl single photon emission tomography: comparison with nitrogen-13 ammonia positron emission tomography. *J Nucl Med* 29:1181–1188, 1988.

15. Demer LL, Gould KL, Goldstein RA, et al: Assessment of coronary artery disease severity by positron emission tomography: comparison with quantitative coronary arteriography in 193 patients. *Circulation* 79:825–835, 1989.

16. Go RT, Marwick TH, MacIntyre WJ, et al: A prospective comparison of rubidium-82 PET and thallium-210 SPECT myocardial perfusion imaging utilizing a single dipyridamole stress in the diagnosis of coronary artery disease. *J Nucl Med* 31:1899–1905, 1990.

17. Stewart RE, Schwaiger M, Molina E, et al: Comparison of rubidium-82 positron emission tomography and thallium-201 SPECT imaging for detection of coronary artery disease. *Am J Cardiol* 67:1303–1310, 1991.

18. Brown KA: Prognostic value of thallium-201 myocardial perfusion imaging: a diagnostic tool comes of age. *Circulation* 83:364–381, 1991.

19. Brown BG, Zhao XQ, Sacco DE, et al: Lipid lowering and plaque regression: new insights into prevention of plaque disruption and clinical events in coronary artery disease. *Circulation* 87:1781–1791, 1993.

20. Gould KL, Martucci JP, Goldberg DI, et al: Short-term cholesterol lowering decreases size and severity of perfusion abnormalities by positron emission tomography after dipyridamole in patients with coronary artery disease. A potential non-invasive marker of healing coronary endothelium. *Circulation* 89:1530–1538, 1994.

21. Gould KL, Ornish D, Scherwitz L, et al: Changes in myocardial perfusion abnormalities by positron emission tomography after long-term, intense risk factor modification. *JAMA* 274:894–901, 1995.

22. Grambow D, Dayanikli F, Muzik O, et al: Assessment of endothelial function with PET cold pressor test in patients with various degrees of coronary atheriosclerosis. *J Nucl Med* 34:36P, 1993.

23. Dayanikli F, Grambow D, Muzik O, et al: Evaluation of coronary flow reserve in asymptomatic males with hyperlipidemia and family history of coronary artery disease. *J Nucl Med* 34:115, 1993.

24. Bergmann SR, Herrero P, Markham J, et al: Noninvasive quantitation of myocardial blood flow in human subjects with oxygen-15-labeled water and positron emission tomography. *J Am Coll Cardiol* 14:639–652, 1989.

25. Hutchins GD, Schwaiger M, Rosenspire KC, et al: Noninvasive quantification of regional blood flow in the human heart using N-13-ammonia and dynamic positron emission tomographic imaging. *J Am Coll Cardiol* 15:1032–1042, 1990.

26. Czernin J, Muller P, Chan S, et al: Influence of age and hemodynamics on myocardial blood flow and flow reserve. *Circulation* 88:62–69, 1993.

27. Krivokapich J, Stevenson LW, Kobashigawa J, et al: Quantification of absolute myocardial perfusion at rest and during exercise with positron emission tomography after human cardiac transplantation. *J Am Coll Cardiol* 18:512–517, 1991.

28. Beanlands RSB, Melon PG, Muzik O, et al: N-13 ammonia PET identifies reduced perfusion reserve in angiographically normal regions of patients with CAD. *Circulation* 86:1–184, 1992.

29. Krivokapich J, Huang SC, Selin CE, et al: Fluorodeoxyglucose rate constants, lumped constant, and glucose metabolic rate in rabbit heart. *Am J Physiol* 252:H777–H787, 1987.

30. Ratib O, Phelps ME, Huang SC, et al: Positron emission tomography with deoxyglucose for estimating local myocardial glucose metabolism. *J Nucl Med* 23:577–586, 1982.

31. Schon H, Schelbert HR, Najafi A, et al: C-11-labeled palmitic acid for noninvasive evaluation of regional myocardial fatty acid metabolism with positron computed tomography. II. Kinetics of C-11-palmitic acid in acutely ischemic myocardium. *Am Heart J* 1103:548–561, 1982.

32. Schelbert HR, Henze E, Schon H, et al: C-11-labeled palmitic acid for noninvasive evaluation of regional myocardial fatty acid metabolism with positron computed tomography.

III. In vivo demonstration of the effects of substrate availability on myocardial metabolism. *Am Heart J* 105:492–504, 1983.

33. Sobel BE, Geltman EM, Tiefenbrunn AJ, et al: Improvement of regional myocardial metabolism after coronary thrombolysis induced with tissue-type plasminogen activator or streptokinase. *Circulation* 69:983–990, 1984.

34. Bergmann SR, Lerch RA, Fox KAA, et al: Temporal dependence of beneficial effects of coronary thrombolysis characterized by positron emission tomography. *Am J Med* 73:573–581, 1982.

35. Knabb RM, Bergmann SR, Fox KAA, et al: The temporal pattern of recovery of myocardial perfusion and metabolism delineated by positron emission tomography following coronary thrombolysis. *J Nucl Med* 28:1563–1570, 1987.

36. Schelbert HR, Henze E, Schon H, et al: C-11-labeled palmitic acid for noninvasive evaluation of regional myocardial fatty acid metabolism with positron computed tomography. III. In vivo demonstration of the effects of substrate availability on myocardial metabolism. *Am Heart J.* 105:492–504, 1983.

37. Schon H, Schelbert HR, Najafi A, et al: C-11-labeled palmitic acid for noninvasive evaluation of regional myocardial fatty acid metabolism with positron computed tomography. II. Kinetics of C-11-palmitic acid in acutely ischemic myocardium. *Am Heart J* 1103:548–561, 1982.

38. Brown M, Myears D, Bergmann S: Validity of estimates of myocardial oxidative metabolism with carbon-11-acetate and positron emission tomography despite altered patterns of substrate utilization. *J Nucl Med* 30:187–193, 1989.

39. Brown M, Marshall D, Sobel B, Delineation of myocardial oxygen utilization with carbon-11-labeled acetate. *Circulation* 76:687–696, 1987.

40. Brown M, Myears D, Bergmann S: Noninvasive assessment of canine myocardial oxidative metabolism with carbon-11-acetate and positron emission tomography. *J Am Coll Cardiol* 12:1054–1063, 1988.

41. Walsh M, Geltman E, Brown M, et al: Noninvasive estimation of regional myocardial oxygen consumption by positron emission tomography with carbon-11-acetate in patients with myocardial infarction. *J Nucl Med* 30:1798–1808, 1989.

42. Buxton DB, Nienaber Ca, Luxen A, et al: Noninvasive quantitation of regional myocardial oxygen consumption in vivo with [1-11C] acetate and dynamic positron emission tomography. *Circulation* 79:134–142, 1989.

43. Armbrecht JJ, Buxton DB, Schelbert HR: Validation of [1-^{11}C] acetate kinetics as a tracer for noninvasive assessment of oxidative metabolism with positron emission tomography in normal, ischemic, postischemic, and hyperemic canine myocardium. *Circulation* 81:1594–1605, 1990.

44. Lear JL: Relationship between myocardial clearance rates of carbon-11-acetate-derived radiolabeled and oxidative metabolism: physiologic basis and clinical significance (editorial). *J Nucl Med* 32:1957–1960, 1991.

45. Marshall RC, Tillisch JH, Phelps ME, et al: Identification and differentiation of resting myocardial ischemia in man with positron computed tomography, 18F-labeled flurodeoxyglucose and N-13-ammonia. *Circulation* 67:766–778, 1983.

46. Tillisch J, Brunken R, Marshall R, et al: Reversibility of cardiac wall-motion abnormalities predicted by positron emission tomography. *N Engl J Med* 314:884–888, 1986.

47. Tamaki N, Yonekura Y, Yamashita K, et al: Positron emission tomography using fluorine-18 deoxyglucose in evaluation of coronary artery bypass grafting. *Am J Cardiol* 64:860–866, 1989.

48. Gropler RJ, Geltman EM, Sampathkumaran K, et al: Functional recovery after coronary revascularization for chronic coronary artery disease is dependent on maintenance of oxidative metabolism. *J Am Coll Cardiol* 20:569–577, 1992.

49. Schwaiger M, Brunken R, Grover-McKay M, et al: Regional myocardial metabolism in patients with acute myocardial infarction assessed by positron emission tomography. *J Am Coll Cardiol* 8:800–808, 1986.

50. Pierard LA, De Landsheere CM, Berthe C, et al: Identification of viable myocardium by echocardiography during dobutamine infusion in patients with myocardial infarction after thrombolytic therapy: comparison with positron emission tomography. *J Am Coll Cardiol* 15:1021–1031, 1990.

51. Tamaki N, Yonekura Y, Yamashita K, et al: Prognostic significance of augmented uptake of FDG on PET in the areas of myocardial infarction. *J Nucl Med* 32:1039, 1991.

52. Eitzman D, Al-Aouar Z, Kanter H, et al: Clinical outcome of patients with advanced coronary artery disease after viability studies with positron emission tomography. *J Am Coll Cardiol* 20:559, 1992.

53. Maddahi J, DiCarli M, Davidson M, et al: Prognostic significance of PET assessment of myocardial viability in patients with left ventricular dysfunction. *J Am Coll Cardiol* 19:142, 1992.

54. Fox KA, Abendschein DR, Ambos HD, et al: Efflux of metabolized and nonmetabolized fatty acid from canine myocardium. Implications for quantifying myocardium metabolism tomographically. *Circ Res* 57:232–243, 1985.

55. Rosamond TL, Abendschein DR, Sobel B, et al: Metabolic fate of radiolabeled palmitate in ischemic canine myocardium: implications for positron emission tomography. *J Nucl Med* 28:1322–1329, 1987.

56. Buxton DB, Mody FV, Krivokapich J, et al: Quantitative assessment of prolonged metabolic abnormalities in reperfused myocardium. *Circulation* 85:1842–1856, 1992.

57. Henes CG, Bergmann SR, Perez JE, et al: The time course of restoration of nutritive perfusion, myocardial oxygen consumption, and regional function after coronary thrombolysis. *Coron Artery Dis* 1:687–696, 1990.

58. Buxton DB, Mody FV, Krivokapich J, et al: Quantitative assessment of prolonged metabolic abnormalities in reperfused myocardium. *Circulation* 85:1842–1856, 1992.

59. Gropler RJ, Siegel BA, Sampathkumaran K, et al: Dependence of recovery of contractile function on maintenance of oxidative metabolism after myocardial infarction. *J Am Coll Cardiol* 19:989–997, 1992.

60. Vanoverschelde J-LJ, Melin JA, Bol A, et al: Regional oxidative metabolism in patients after recovery from reperfused anterior myocardial infarction: relation to regional blood flow and glucose uptake. *Circulation* 85:9–21, 1992.

61. Yamamoto Y, de Silva R, Rhodes CG, et al: A new strategy for assessment of viable myocardium and regional myocardial blood flow using ^{15}O-water and dynamic positron emission tomography. *Circulation* 86:167–178, 1992.

62. Schwaiger M, Kalff V, Rosenspire K, et al: Noninvasive evaluation of sympathetic nervous system in the human heart by positron emission tomography. *Circulation* 82:457, 1990.

63. Goldstein DS, Chang PC, Eisenhofer G, et al: Positron emission tomographic imaging of cardiac sympathetic innervation and function. *Circulation* 1606–1621, 1990.

64. Kinsey BM, Barber R, Tewson TJ: Synthesis of fluorine-18 fluorocarazolol, a high affinity ligand for the β-adrenergic receptor (abstract). *J Nucl Med* 33:983, 1992.

65. Zheng L, Berridge MS: [18F]Fluorocarazolol: a potential beta-adrenergic radiotracer for PET (abstract). *J Nucl Med* 33:984, 1992.

66. Maziere M, Comar D, Godot JM, et al: In vivo characterization of myocardium muscarinic receptors by positron emission tomography. *Life Sci* 29:2391–2397, 1981.

67. Charbonneau P, Syrota A, Crouzel C, et al: Peripheral-type benzodiazepine receptors in the living heart characterized by positron emission tomography. *Circulation* 73:476–483, 1986.

68. Ehrin E, Luthra SK, Crouzel C, et al: Preparation of carbon-11 labeled prazosin, a potent and selective α_1-adrenergic antagonist. *J Label Compds Radiopharm* 25:177–183, 1988.

69. Lemaire C, Cantineau R, Guillaume M, et al: Fluorine-18-Altanserin: a radioligand for the study of serotonin receptors with PET: radiolabeling and the in vivo biologic behavior in rats. *J Nucl Med* 91:2266–2272, 1991.

70. Ficaro EP, Fressler JA, Shreve PD, et al: Simultaneous transmission/emission myocardial perfusion tomography: diagnostic accuracy of attenuated-corrected Tc-99m sestamibi single-photon emission tomography. *Circulation* 93:463–473, 1996.

71. Patterson RE, Eisner RL, Horowitz SF: Comparison of cost-effectiveness and utility of exercise ECG, single photon emission tomography, and coronary artery angiography for diagnosis of coronary artery disease. *Circulation* 91:54–65, 1995.

—4—

Magnetic Resonance Imaging

Roxann Rokey, M.D.
G. Wesley Vick, M.D.

DESCRIPTION OF TECHNIQUE

Magnetic resonance imaging (MRI) techniques use the principles of nuclear magnetic resonance and digital imaging technology to generate a variety of clinically useful types of images. Great progress in the application of MRI to neurologic and orthopedic imaging problems has been made since the inception of MRI in the early 1970s. The application of MRI to cardiovascular assessment, though technically difficult because of cardiac and respiratory motion, has also substantially advanced. Cardiovascular MRI is a complex method that requires the availability of sophisticated instrumentation. This instrumentation includes a magnet to provide a large static magnetic field, radiofrequency pulse and electromagnetic gradient coil subsystems to facilitate spatial localization of magnetic resonance signal, computers to control data acquisition and process images, and hardware to enable synchronization of image acquisition with the cardiac cycle. In order to provide clinically relevant information, physicians acquiring and interpreting MRI studies should have a sound working knowledge of the technique as well as expertise in cardiovascular anatomy and physiology and the clinical course of disease processes.

DEVELOPMENTAL PERSPECTIVES

Mass, energy, and all of their properties are ultimately discrete rather than continuous. This phenomenon is known as quantization. Quantization of atomic nuclear magnetic moments provides the fundamental basis for the nuclear magnetic resonance phenomenon, and was first demonstrated by Gerlach and Stern in the 1920s. In 1946, Bloch and Purcell, working independently, discovered that under proper conditions, atomic nuclei in a magnetic field would produce a radiofrequency signal that could be detected by an appropriately designed radio antenna and receiver. Nuclear magnetic resonance devices soon became indispensable in analytic organic chemistry for evaluation of molecular structure. However, the technique remained time-consuming. This changed in 1966 when Ernst described the use of pulsed magnetic resonance in conjunction with Fourier transformation in nuclear magnetic resonance experiments.[1] Ernst's method greatly speeded the acquisition of magnetic resonance data and made additional developments feasible. The concept of MRI was proposed by Damadian in a patent application filed in 1972. However, the first MRI (two tubes of water) was published in *Nature* by Lauterbur in 1973.[2] The images were created by resonance localization with magnetic field gradients. This concept is employed today, with various modifications, in nearly all MRI systems. In 1976, Damadian and colleagues published the first MRI image of the thorax of a living human.[3] Cardiac and vascular motion initially precluded useful MRI evaluations of the heart. However, in the early 1980s, when hardware and software were developed to allow acquisition of images in synchrony with the cardiac cycle, practical cardiovascular MRI became feasible. In the last decade, cardiovascular MRI has been tested and refined. It can provide practical and valuable information and is the imaging technique of choice in a number of clinical situations.

TECHNICAL CONSIDERATIONS

Commercially available clinical MRI units are large devices that occupy one or more rooms and usually require special shielding to reduce interference from environmental electromagnetic fields and ensure that fringe magnetic fields from the central magnet will be contained within the MRI unit. Typically MRI scanners are used to evaluate multiple organ systems. Only a few dedicated cardiovascular MRI systems are operational at this time. It follows that in many practice situations there are limitations on the MRI imaging time available for cardiovascular studies. In many cases, MRI technologists have the responsibility for actual acquisition of the MRI studies. Substantial additional training of general MRI technologists is usually necessary before they can be expected to perform good quality cardiovascular examinations. Our experience has been that in cardiovascular problems of significant complexity, close supervision by knowledgeable physicians during the study is invaluable. A nurse who can administer sedatives to young children and potentially claustrophobic patients is helpful in order to facilitate patient throughput and maximize physician utilization.

All conventional MRI units suitable for cardiovascular examinations contain six major components. These are:

1. the magnet
2. the computer
3. the radiofrequency transmitter
4. the radiofrequency receiver
5. the gradient coil system
6. the physiologic monitoring and synchronization system (ECG, pulse oximeter, respiratory gating equipment)

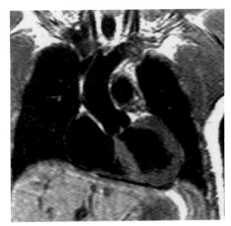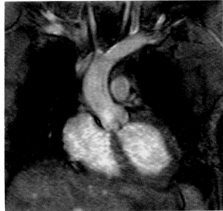

Figure 4.1. Coronal MRI of the heart at the same anatomic level obtained using two different imaging techniques. The image on the left acquired with a spin-echo technique ("black-blood" method) demonstrates myocardium and blood vessel walls with high signal intensity compared to the blood vessel lumen and cardiac chamber cavities. The image on the right acquired with the gradient echo technique ("bright blood" technique or "cine" MRI) shows the myocardium and blood vessel walls with relatively low signal intensity while the blood vessel lumen and cardiac chamber cavities contain high signal intensity.

A thorough knowledge of the physics and instrumentation involved in the generation of cardiovascular MRI is crucial for the physician supervising and interpreting the study. For the physician ordering the test, familiarity with only a few general concepts is essential. The most important concept is that contrast between flowing blood and the myocardial and blood vessel walls provides the basis for cardiovascular MRI. The second important concept is that two general types of MRI technique can be used to provide this contrast (Figure 4.1):

1. Spin-echo technique
2. Gradient echo technique

Images obtained with the spin-echo technique demonstrate the myocardium and blood vessel walls with a relatively high signal intensity, while the blood vessel lumens and cardiac chamber cavities are shown with a relatively low signal intensity. Thus, the spin-echo technique, as it is usually implemented, is a "black-blood" method.

Images obtained with standard gradient echo imaging sequences demonstrate the myocardium and blood vessel walls with a relatively low signal intensity, whereas the blood vessel lumens and cardiac chamber cavities are shown with a relatively high signal intensity. Thus, the gradient echo technique, as it is usually implemented, is a "bright-blood" technique. When gradient echo images are acquired at multiple points in the cardiac cycle and displayed in continuous loop format, the resultant digital movies are termed "cine" MRI, since they are similar in appearance to the angiographic standard.

A third concept is that image contrast can be substantially altered by the specific implementation of the spin-echo or gradient echo technique. Manipulation of imaging parameters is an important tool for delineating anatomic structures of interest and defining pathologic features.

A fourth important concept is that MRI images are usually acquired over multiple cardiac and respiratory cycles. It follows that cardiovascular MRI image quality is critically dependent on the presence of a stable heart rate and on respirations that are regular and not of excessive amplitude. Furthermore, since image acquisition requires a relatively long time, substantial voluntary or involuntary patient motions during the acquisition can have major deleterious effects on the images. Recently developed rapid MRI imaging methods substantially reduce the motion artifacts that can degrade MRI images.

INDICATIONS AND USES

Although multiple applications of cardiovascular MRI have been described in the last decade, many of these applications remain investigational at the present time. However, in the four disease categories indicated in Table 4.1, cardiovascular MRI is no longer considered investigational and has become a part of standard clinical practice in many localities. The frequency with which an individual physician will have reason to request a cardiovascular MRI study will, of course, depend on the number of patients that he or she evaluates in these disease categories. For physicians primarily dealing with adult patients, the most common indication for requesting a cardiovascular MRI study is to evaluate known or suspected acquired aortic disease, such as aortic aneurysm and/or aortic dissection. With MRI, rapid and precise assessment of the entire aorta can be performed noninvasively and without use of ionizing radiation or iodinated contrast. For physicians who frequently see patients with congenital heart disease, cardiovascular MRI is primarily used to assess congenital malformations. The features of complex congenital cardiovascular disorders can be clearly demonstrated with MRI, which is complementary to echocardiography and surpasses this technique as well as angiography in certain diagnostic categories. Pericardial disease is relatively common in both adult and pediatric cardiology practices. The imaging diagnosis of pericardial effusion is readily made with echocardiography, but in those unusual cases where pericardial constriction is suspected, MRI can define pericardial thickness, which is difficult to assess by echocardiography. Paracardiac masses are uncommonly seen. When these masses are suspected, MRI is usually superior to echocardiography and computed tomography for assessment, and can provide valuable information about their size, location, and character.

TABLE 4.1. Indications for Cardiovascular MRI

1. Great vessel disease
2. Complex congenital disease
3. Pericardial disease
4. Cardiac and paracardiac masses

Great Vessel Disease

Aortic Aneurysms

Aneurysms of the thoracic and abdominal aorta are readily delineated with nuclear magnetic resonance (NMR) imaging. Although standard x-ray contrast angiography, ultrasonography, and x-ray computed tomography can also demonstrate aortic aneurysms, MRI has the advantages of being noninvasive, of not employing ionizing radiation, of not requiring intravenous contrast, of not being impeded by poor ultrasonic windows, and of facilitating acquisition of tomographic sections or three-dimensional projections of the aorta in any desired orientation. Precise measurements of aortic luminal diameter can easily be obtained from MRI images and serial evaluations of aneurysm size are readily made.

Aortic Dissection

A variety of noninvasive and invasive imaging techniques have been used in the evaluation of aortic dissection. These include MRI, echocardiography, and computed tomography and angiography. When appraising patients with suspected or known dissection, three important questions arise:

1. Is there a dissection of the aorta?
2. Is the ascending aorta involved?
3. What other information is needed to manage the case?

Regardless of the imaging modality, demonstration of an intimal flap and double lumen are specific findings that allow confident diagnosis of a dissection. Definition of the entry and exit site to the false lumen is helpful since definitive surgery at most centers consists of excision of the entry site, obliteration of the exit site, and replacement of the involved aorta where possible. Additionally, when aortic arch involvement is suspected, evaluation of aortic arch vessels is imperative. Because MRI has a wide field of view involving the ascending aorta, aortic arch, and descending aorta in addition to the arch vessels and is capable of producing both anatomic images and multiphasic images of blood flow, it is well suited for the diagnosis of aortic dissection (Figure 4.2). In comparison with computed tomography, transesophageal echocardiography, transthoracic echocardiography, better visualization of the arch vessels, and fewer false-negative and false-positive findings have been reported.[4–6] MRI is safe, specific, and sensitive in the assessment of acute and chronic dissection when performed and interpreted by experienced observers. The same also applies in the postoperative evaluation of surgically repaired dissection.

The major limitation of MRI in dissection assessment is related to the technical aspects of dealing with acutely ill patients. Although there is no impediment to hemodynamic, respiratory, or electrocardiographic monitoring in the magnet, patients must necessarily be moved to the MRI imaging suite and positioned in the magnet bore. When patients are positioned for imaging, access to them is limited. Investigational studies have demonstrated that MRI can be safely performed in patients with acute infarction and acute aortic dissection.[7,8] Despite these findings, there is at the present time a reluctance to perform MRI studies in acutely ill patients.

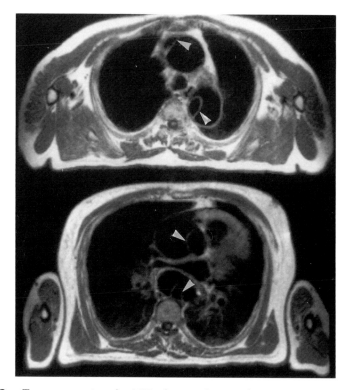

Figure 4.2.   Transverse spin-echo MRI of a type I aortic dissection obtained at two different anatomic levels (upper and lower panel). The ascending aorta is located anteriorly and the
descending aorta posteriorly in both panels. The intimal flap (white arrowheads) with double
lumen in the ascending and descending aorta are both clearly delineated at each anatomic
level.

Improvements in magnet design and imaging speed promise to facilitate MRI in
acute aortic dissection.

Intramural hematoma of the thoracic aorta has recently been described. With
this disorder, no evidence of double lumen or intimal disruption is found, although
extensive wall thickening is caused by the hematoma. The rupture of the vasa vaso-
rum may be the initiating event leading to intramural hematoma. Ultimately, the
presence of hematoma may lead to frank aortic dissection. MRI can clearly demonstrate aortic intramural hematoma.[9] Such hematomas may be missed by angiography.

Vascular Rings

A variety of congenital malformations of the aortic arch occur. Some of these are
primarily of academic interest, but in a group of these anomalies, the esophagus and
trachea are completely encircled by vascular tissue, forming a "vascular ring". If the
vascular ring is loose, it will cause no difficulty. However, if the vascular tissue com-
presses the trachea and esophagus, it will cause stridor and/or dysphagia. The most
common types of vascular ring are variants of double aortic arch and of right aortic
arch with retroesophageal left subclavian artery. MRI is an ideal imaging tool for

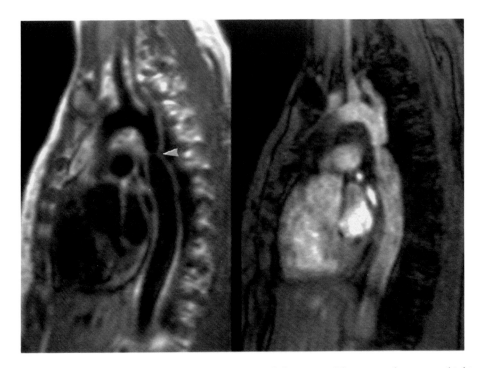

Figure 4.3. MRI of a patient with coarctation of the aorta. The spin-echo image (right panel) demonstrates the coarctation in the descending thoracic aorta (arrowhead). The gradient echo image (left panel) provides an image similar to the cineangiographic standard.

defining vascular rings, because it clearly depicts the relationship of the trachea and esophagus to the anomalous aortic arch vessels.

Coarctation of the Aorta

A considerable body of experience has demonstrated the utility of MRI in the evaluation of coarctation of the aorta, both before and after treatment (Figure 4.3). The presence of stenosis at a discrete coarctation site can be detected and the diameter and length of narrowed aortic segments can be assessed as well as the presence of post-stenotic dilation. MRI can also detect aneurysms that occur after coarctation surgery or balloon dilation.[10,11] Collateral vessels may be visualized on MRI studies of patients with coarctation and hemodynamically substantial obstruction to blood flow. Cine MRI angiographic techniques are useful for evaluating the hemodynamic importance of obstruction to blood flow at the coarctation site and in assessing the adequacy of collateral formation.

Marfan's Syndrome

Evaluation of Marfan's syndrome by MRI has also been well described. The aorta in Marfan's syndrome is characteristically enlarged in the region of the sinuses of Valsalva in relation to other portions of the aorta. Kerstine-Sommerhoff and colleagues found that the ratio of aortic diameter at the sinuses of Valsalva to diameter in the upper descending aorta was 1.4 or greater with Marfan's syndrome and 1.3 or less in patients with other causes of aortic enlargement and in normals.[12] MRI is an excellent tool for quantifying aortic enlargement in this disorder, ruling out aortic dissection, and monitoring the results of operative therapy for aortic aneurysmal dilation.

Congenital Heart Disease

Improved medical and surgical treatment of congenital heart disease has resulted in an increased survival of infants with complex congenital heart disease. As a result, the number of adolescents and adults with complex lesions is increasing. Consideration of palliative and/or corrective procedures for complex lesions requires full preoperative anatomic and hemodynamic assessment of the underlying lesion. Followup of such patients requires assessment of any persistent postoperative residual anatomic lesions, the success of palliative or corrective procedures, and any complications of surgical or interventional procedures.

It is beyond the scope of this chapter to describe the myriad of congenital cardiac lesions and the palliative and corrective procedures that have been developed for their treatment. Many of these congenital anomalies are rarely encountered in routine clinical practice. Imaging evaluations of these disorders are best performed by physicians who have had extensive training in the assessment of congenital heart disease and require an individualized approach that is addressed to specific clinical questions.

Echocardiography remains the primary noninvasive method for initial evaluation of complex congenital heart disease. However, in some infants, and in many older children and adults, echocardiographic visualization of clinically important cardiovascular structures is severely impaired because of poor ultrasonic penetration. In these patients, MRI is an important adjunctive procedure which is complementary to the echocardiographic assessment.[13,14]

Because of its wide field of view and excellent soft tissue contrast, MRI is an excellent tool for evaluation of complex congenital cardiovascular disease. The visceral and cardiac situs is readily apparent on MRI. The atrioventricular and ventriculoarterial connections are usually easily discerned. Delineation of great vessel anatomy and its relationship to other structures is an important strength of MRI. The ascending and descending aorta, the distal pulmonary arteries, and the pulmonary and systemic veins are well defined by MRI. Major aortopulmonary collateral vessels can be clearly demonstrated, as can the right ventricular cavity and the right ventricular anterior wall. These structures are of particular importance in many varieties of congenital heart disease and are not adequately visualized after infancy by echocardiography in many patients. Although transesophageal echocardiography is often useful in these patients because of its clear delineation of intracardiac anatomy, transesophageal echocardiography does not typically visualize many important extracardiac structures with the clarity of MRI. Furthermore, transesophageal echocardiography is more invasive, and requires a substantially greater degree of sedation in most pediatric and adolescent patients than does MRI.

MRI is very helpful in evaluation of results of palliative operations such as the modified Blalock-Taussig shunt, the Glenn shunt, and pulmonary artery banding.

MRI is also useful in the assessment of corrective operations such as tetralogy of Fallot repair, the modified Fontan procedure, the Jatene procedure, and Rastelli conduit operations. Again, echocardiographic evaluation alone often fails to adequately delineate important cardiovascular features in patients who have undergone these operations.[14]

Pericardial Disease

Pericarditis with subsequent pericardial effusion or pericardial thickening involving the parietal or visceral pericardium may be caused by a number of different etiologies. The anatomic manifestations of acute pericarditis, pericardial thickening, and pericardial fibrosis/calcification are demonstrable with a variety of noninvasive techniques, including echocardiography, MRI, and computed tomography.

Echocardiography remains the noninvasive procedure of choice in diagnosis of pericardial effusion. However, cardiac MRI can provide the following additional information when clinically necessary:

1. Detection of small effusions strongly suspected but not demonstrated with ultrasound
2. Visualization of loculated pericardial effusions
3. Differentiating pericardial from pleural effusions
4. Characterizing the composition of fluid

Although computed tomography can also provide some of this additional information, MRI is superior for characterization of the composition of pericardial fluid. Initial detection of pericardial effusion is accomplished with spin-echo MRI. By manipulating the parameters in the spin-echo sequence, if the effusion is moderate to large in size, the effusion can be defined as transudative, exudative, hemorrhagic, or lipoid in composition.[15,16]

Pericardial thickening, a hallmark of pericardial constriction, is well demonstrated with MRI.[17,18] Pericardial thickness is overestimated with both MRI and computed tomography techniques. However, in such cases, using MRI, small pericardial effusions can be differentiated from thickened and fibrotic and/or calcified pericardium using the spin-echo and gradient echo techniques. With spin-echo images the effusion and thickened pericardium appear dark. Using cine MRI, effusions will become bright, consistent with mobile fluid, whereas the thickened and fibrotic and/or calcified pericardium will remain dark. The process of pericardial constriction most likely represents a continuous process until the pericardium ultimately fibroses or calcifies. Thus, using the MRI technique, it is also possible to infer the diagnosis of effusive constrictive pericardial process when the presence of a thickened pericardium with either mobile or nonmobile fluid is detected (Figure 4.4). Using MRI, the diagnosis of constrictive pericarditis may also be construed indirectly from associated anatomic findings such as dilated systemic veins and relatively small ventricular cavity size. Quantitative assessment of intracardiac flows and pressures is also helpful in establishing the diagnosis of constrictive pericarditis. This flow and pressure information is usually acquired by cardiac catheterization or echocardiography, but could potentially be obtained by MRI.

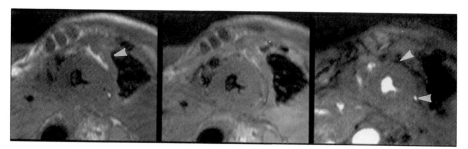

Figure 4.4. MRI of a patient with effusive constrictive pericarditis following cardiac surgery. The short axis spin-echo image (left panel) of the heart shows the left ventricle surrounded by a thickened pericardium anteriorly and laterally (white arrowhead). The white substance immediately adjacent to the left ventricle indicates a nonfibrotic component. The later spin-echo image (middle panel) also shows a thickened pericardium but differentiation of thickened versus nonfibrotic substance is not possible. The gradient echo image (right panel) indicates that there is persistent thickened pericardium and both mobile and nonmobile fluid (arrowheads).

Cardiac and Paracardiac Masses

With a wide field of view and excellent soft tissue contrast, MRI is well suited to evaluation of intra- and extracardiac masses (Figure 4.5).[19] It is preferable to echocardiography in defining the latter and is superior to computed tomography in assessing the extent and effect of mediastinal masses on adjacent cardiovascular structures. Spin-echo anatomic images provide information about the location and extent of invasion of the mass into the pericardial space or other cardiac structures. In addition the spin-echo images can often be used to characterize the mass. Lipomas and thickened pericardial fat pads have a characteristic high signal intensity on appropriately timed spin-echo imaging sequences. Pericardial cysts typically have a low internal signal intensity on certain spin-echo sequences and a homogenous high signal intensity on other types of spin-echo sequences. Cardiac and paracardiac tumors typically show enhanced signal intensity subsequent to infusion of MRI contrast agents such as gadolinium diethylenetriamine penta-acetic acid (DTPA). The signal intensity of thrombus, on the other hand, is not increased by MRI contrast agents. Cine MRI can demonstrate the degree of motility of intracardiac masses during the cardiac cycle and can delineate the dynamic consequences of extrinsic masses on cardiac contraction.

CONTRAINDICATIONS

Implanted metallic objects are a subject of concern. Such objects could potentially undergo undesirable torquing movements if the magnetic field is sufficiently strong and if they contain sufficient ferromagnetic material. Surgical clips and sternotomy wires implanted in the chest and abdomen are weakly ferromagnetic and quickly become immobilized by surrounding fibrous tissue. Hence, patients with these

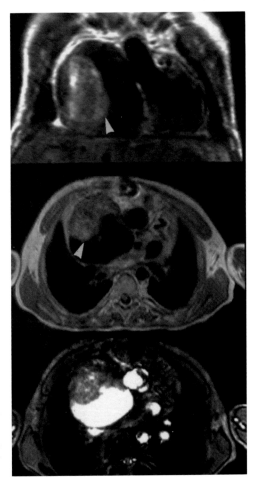

Figure 4.5. MRI of large right atrial thrombus in a patient with a classic Fontan procedure (right atrium to pulmonary artery connection) for tricuspid atresia. The mass was not well delineated by echocardiographic means. The coronal spin-echo image (top panel) shows the large right mass extending the length of the right atrium (arrowhead). The transverse spin-echo (middle panel) also shows the width of the mass. The gradient echo image (lower panel) demonstrates that there is some blood flow within the mass in addition to expected blood flow within the remainder of the atrium.

implants can be routinely studied. Intracranial aneurysm clips do not become immobilized by fibrous tissue, however, and can undergo torque in a magnetic field. Although nonferromagnetic aneurysm clips are available now, MRI studies of patients with these intracranial clips are contraindicated unless the clip is specifically known to be nonferromagnetic. Other types of intracranial ferromagnetic objects or materials may also contraindicate MRI studies. Welders are prone to accidents that may result in the intracranial implantation of potentially mobile ferromagnetic chips.

Prosthetic cardiac valves manufactured after 1964 contain little ferromagnetic material and patients with these valves can be studied safely. On the other hand, heart valves manufactured before 1964 may contain substantial amounts of ferromagnetic material, and MRI study of patients with these implants may be contraindicated. Fortunately, the number of patients with these early valves still in place is very small.

The presence of a cardiac pacemaker is a contraindication to MRI studies, mainly because of concern that the pacemaker electronics might be damaged. It is also possible that magnetic field gradients could induce currents in the pacemaker leads and that these currents could be recognized as cardiac activity by the electronic sensing mechanisms of the pacemaker. The pacemaker might then be improperly inhibited. Another possibility is that the reed switch of the pacemaker could be activated, causing it to pace in the asynchronous mode.

ADVANTAGES AND DISADVANTAGES

MRI can provide anatomic and functional information of superb quality in a variety of cardiovascular imaging applications noninvasively and without exposing patients to ionizing radiation. Thus there is no question that MRI has significant advantages in selected clinical situations.

However, MRI does have some inherent disadvantages. MRI is capital-intensive, requiring a large investment in an expensive scanner and support facilities. The operating costs of most MRI units are substantial, because of the necessity to replace cryogens, and because significant engineering support is typically necessary to keep the scanner functioning optimally. Furthermore, achieving optimum cardiovascular MRI studies requires that the individuals responsible for performing and interpreting the studies have high levels of expertise in cardiovascular pathophysiology, in MRI technique, and in digital imaging methods. Thus, the need for skilled personnel is high. It follows that MRI is necessarily an expensive imaging technique, although actual patient charges for MRI compare very favorably with invasive imaging and are similar to those associated with nuclear cardiology techniques. Another consideration is convenience: MRI examinations at present are relatively lengthy. They require that the patient be moved to the imaging suite and placed in a confined space. Some patients may be claustrophobic and may object to the noise that is associated with MRI imaging. Patients with pacemakers cannot be studied with MRI at the present time.

Echocardiography and computed tomography are the two competing noninvasive methods that have been used in the diagnosis of the disease categories described. Angiography and hemodynamic measurements have also been widely used in evaluation of these disease categories. Because echocardiographic equipment has a relatively low capital cost and because the equipment is portable, it is likely that echocardiography will continue to be the initial imaging modality in many of these cases. When echocardiography fails to supply necessary information for clinical decisions, other techniques will be employed to obtain the required data. The suitability of MRI in any particular situation will depend on the patient characteristics, the expertise and facilities available, and on the specific questions that need to be answered.

SPECIAL CONSIDERATIONS

Approximately 90% of a medical cardiologist's practice is devoted to management of patients with atherosclerotic cardiovascular disease. Although MRI is being widely utilized for diagnosis of aortic disease, MRI applications in atherosclerotic coronary artery disease have been limited to a few specialized centers. Assessments of myocardial mass, regional wall motion, left and right ventricular ejection fractions, cardiac volumetric flows, pressure gradients, and valvular function are all possible now with MRI. The data obtained compare favorably with other invasive and non-invasive tests. Indeed, MRI evaluation of ventricular mass and ejection fraction is considered by many to be the "gold standard" for these measurements. Further technical enhancements promise to make cardiovascular MRI more reliable and easier to perform.

However, echocardiography and nuclear medicine have provided this information for years, and the necessary facilities and personnel for providing echocardiographic and nuclear cardiology studies are widely available. In order for MRI to replace these techniques for the assessment of atherosclerotic coronary artery disease in general clinical practice, it will be necessary for MRI to show a comparatively superior cost/benefit relationship in large-scale studies. Limited access to magnets, limited ability of cardiovascular specialists to perform and interpret MRI studies, and limited funding for health care are likely to restrict use of cardiovascular MRI for commonly performed assessments of ischemic cardiovascular disease in the foreseeable future. However, if noninvasive MRI coronary angiographic techniques are shown to be accurate and relatively inexpensive compared to the invasive standard (see below), cardiovascular MRI may take a prominent position in the diagnosis and management of coronary artery disease.

FUTURE ADVANCEMENT

Anatomic delineation of native coronary artery anatomy and coronary artery bypass grafts is now possible with MRI.[20,21] However, further refinement of MRI coronary angiography will be necessary before it achieves wide clinical usage. Specifically, imaging time must be reduced, cardiorespiratory motion artifact must be substantially decreased, and significant improvements in image resolution must be achieved. Once these problems are dealt with, routine MRI coronary angiography should be possible. Coronary artery flow mapping has also been performed with MRI.[22] Myocardial tagging with MRI is another promising method for myocardial functional evaluation. This technique can provide a multiphasic quantitative three-dimensional picture of myocardial contraction and stress. This information may prove helpful in identifying regions of "hibernating" myocardium and myocardial scar. Several recent studies have demonstrated that myocardial perfusion can be evaluated with MRI, subsequent to intravenous infusion of MRI contrast agents. Finally, interesting investigational work suggests that MRI evaluation of high-energy phosphate metabolism and even myocardial tissue oxygen saturation may become clinically applicable.

SUMMARY

Present cardiovascular MRI techniques provide excellent anatomic and functional detail of the heart and great vessels. Clear indications exist for the application of this technology to patients with known or suspected great vessel disease, complex congenital heart disease, pericardial disease, and cardiac/paracardiac masses. MRI of coronary arteries is now possible. Further refinement of these MRI coronary angiographic techniques will probably enhance its widespread usage and allow this technology to take a prominent role in the diagnosis of cardiovascular atherosclerotic coronary heart disease.

REFERENCES

1. Ernst RR, Anderson WA: Application of Fourier transform spectroscopy to magnetic resonance. *Rev Sci Instrum* 37:93–102, 1966.
2. Lauterbur PC: Image formation by induced local interactions: examples employing nuclear magnetic resonance. *Nature* 242:190–191, 1973.
3. Damadian R, Minkhoff L, Goldsmith M, et al: Field focusing nuclear magnetic resonance (FONAR): visualization of a tumor in a live animal. *Science* 194:1430–1431, 1976.
4. Barbant SD, Eisenberg MJ, Schiller NB: The diagnostic value of imaging techniques for aortic dissection. *Am Heart J* 124:541–543, 1992.
5. Nienaber CA, Spielmann RP, Von Kodolitsch Y, et al: Diagnosis of thoracic aortic dissection. *Circulation* 85:434–447, 1992.
6. Deutsch HJ, Sechtem U, Meyer H, et al: Chronic aortic dissection: comparison of MR imaging and transesophageal echocardiography. *Radiology* 192:645–650, 1994.
7. Panting JR, Norell MS, Baker C, et al: Feasibility, accuracy and safety of magnetic resonance imaging in acute aortic dissection. *Clin Radiol* 50:455–458, 1995.
8. Rokey R, Wendt RE, Johnston DL: Monitoring of acutely ill patients during nuclear magnetic resonance imaging: use of a time-varying filter electrocardiographic gating device to reduce gradient artifacts. *Magn Reson Med* 6(2):240–245, 1988.
9. Robbins RC, McManus RP, Mitchell RS, et al: Management of patients with intramural hematoma of the thoracic aorta. *Circulation* 88(part 2):1–10, 1993.
10. Morrow WR, Vick GW III, Nihill MR, et al: Balloon dilation of unoperated coarctation of the aorta: short and intermediate-term results. *J Am Coll Cardiol* 11:133–138, 1988.
11. Boxer RA, LaCorte MA, Singh S, et al: Nuclear magnetic resonance imaging in evaluation and follow-up of children treated for coarctation of the aorta. *J Am Coll Cardiol* 7:1095–1098, 1986.
12. Kerstin-Sommerhoff BA, Sechtem UP, Shiller, NB, et al: MR imaging of the thoracic aorta in Marfan patients. *J Comput Assist Tomogr* 11:633–639, 1987.
13. Vick GW, Rokey R, Huhta JC, et al: Nuclear magnetic resonance imaging of the pulmonary arteries, subpulmonary region, and aorticopulmonary shunts: a comparative study with two dimensional echocardiography and angiography. *Am Heart J* 119:1103–1110, 1990.
14. Hirsch R, Kilner PJ, Connelly MS, et al: Diagnosis in adolescents and adults with congenital heart disease: prospective assessment of individual and combined roles of magnetic resonance imaging and transesophageal echocardiography. *Circulation* 90:2937–2951, 1994.
15. Rokey R, Vick GW, Bolli RM, et al: Assessment of experimental pericardial effusion using nuclear magnetic resonance imaging techniques. *Am Heart J* 121:1161–11169, 1991.
16. Mulvagh SL, Rokey R, Vick GW, et al: Usefulness of nuclear magnetic resonance imag-

ing for evaluation of pericardial effusions and comparison with two dimensional echocardiography. *Am J Cardiol* 64:1002–1009, 1989.

17. Sechtem U, Tscholakoff D, Higgins CB: MRI of the abnormal pericardium. *Am J Roentgenol* 147:245–252, 1986.

18. Soulen RL, Stark DD, Higgins CB: Magnetic resonance imaging of constrictive pericardial disease. *Am J Cardiol* 55:480–484, 1985.

19. Freedberg RS, Kronzon I, Rumancik WM, et al: The contribution of magnetic resonance imaging to the evaluation of intracardiac tumors diagnosed by echocardiography. *Circulation* 77:96–103, 1988.

20. Manning WJ, Li W, Edelman RR. A preliminary report comparing magnetic resonance coronary angiography with conventional angiography. *N Engl J Med* 328:828–832, 1993.

21. Pennell DJ, Keegan J, Firmain DN, et al: Magnetic resonance imaging of coronary arteries: technique and preliminary results. *Br Heart J* 70:315–326, 1993.

22. Clarke G, Eckels R, Chaney C, et al: Measurement of absolute epicardial coronary artery flow with flow reserve with breath-hold cine phase-contrast magnetic resonance imaging. *Circulation* 91:2627–2634, 1995.

— 5 —

Computed Tomography of the Cardiovascular System

Thomas D. Hedrick, M.D.
John J. Mahmarian, M.D.

DESCRIPTION OF TECHNIQUE

Computed tomography (CT) has served a major role in the evaluation of the aorta since its inception in the early 1970s. Several factors limited the use of CT in the cardiovascular system outside of the aorta; traditional computed tomography is inherently limited to cross-sectional imaging in the axial plane which is not always optimal for vessels that may be oriented longitudinally within the body. The time needed to acquire individual slices generally limits the distance along the body which can be reasonably examined during breath-holding and the passage of contrast material. Thus, the development, in the early 1990s, of the helical CT scanner has overcome many of the obstacles which previously limited CT to the evaluation of simple pathology, such as aortic aneurysms.

The speed of new helical scanners allows as many as 60 slices to be obtained rapidly with excellent spatial resolution. A helical scanner can image the entire thoracic and abdominal aorta in the time required for the passage of intravenous contrast material and during the suspension of respiration. The parallel development of a new type of CT scanner utilizing an electron beam to produce x-rays at an extremely rapid rate now allows CT slices to be acquired in a fraction of the cardiac cycle. Ultrafast scanners are capable of visualizing the human heart in freeze-frame motion, and powerful computer workstations reconfigure the images produced by traditional, helical, and electron beam CT scanners. These special-purpose image manipulators allow a series of CT slices to be reconfigured into multiple imaging planes. Planes and projections simulate a typical angiographic study of the aorta and its major branches produced from a basic set of postcontrast CT data.

Flow and motion studies can be analyzed for images acquired through the human heart to obtain data equivalent to that previously acquired from echocardiography and nuclear cardiology studies. Computed tomography is no longer limited to visualizing the aorta but, in fact, is a powerful tool for the evaluation of various diseases of the aorta, pulmonary artery, vena cava, coronary arteries, and heart chambers.

TECHNICAL CONSIDERATIONS

Traditional CT scanners produce images by rotating an x-ray tube around a circular gantry through which the patient passes on a table. The table moves in an incremental fashion with one slice acquired for each table motion. Generally, each tube rotation results in the creation of one slice of CT data. The time required to acquire each slice is usually in the range of 2 sec, and, with the delay between each scan required for table movement and patient respiration, approximately one slice is produced every 10 sec. Helical CT scanners, also known as spiral or slip-ring scanners, allow the x-ray tube to move continuously around the gantry. The helical CT table moves continuously through the gantry without incremental stops. The CT tube makes its revolution around the patient in 1 sec, and the table can move at the rate of approximately two slices per second through the gantry (Figure 5.1). The helical CT scanner acquires approximately 60 CT slices within a 30-sec breath-hold; these slices may be of any desired thickness (usually 5–10 mm). During two breath-holds,

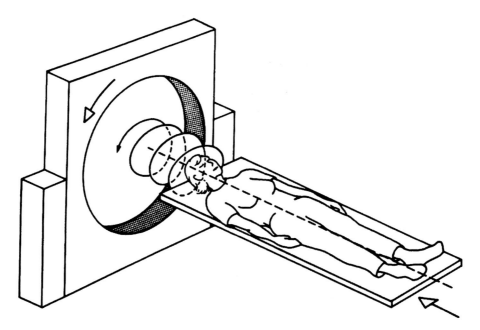

Figure 5.1. Diagram tracing helical (spiral) path of x-ray beam as patient moves continuously through gantry while tube rotates continuously around patient. From Brink JA. Technical Aspects of Helial (Spiral) CT. In: Silverman PM (ed) *Radiol Clin North Am* 33: 1995, 826. Reproduced with permission from W.B. Saunders.

it is quite possible to cover the entire thoracic and abdominal aorta during an overall time of approximately 90 sec. The continuous infusion of iodinated contrast material is accomplished via an injector through a peripheral intravenous site. Excellent contrast CT of the entire aorta and its branches can be obtained easily using the helical technique.[1]

Electron beam CT scanners, also called Ultrafast scanners, use an alternate method of generating the x-ray beam. Rather than sweeping a weighty x-ray tube and its associated electronic equipment around the patient, an electron beam is passed in a circular fashion around the patient. The electron beam is generated by an electron gun positioned behind the gantry and focused with a very controlled magnetic field on four tungsten rings contained in the gantry. As the electrons strike the tungsten ring, x-rays are emitted and collimated to a selected slice thickness (Figure 5.2). The beam of electrons may be swept around the tungsten rings in a circular fashion acquiring a slice in 50 msec. This speed is more than sufficient to enable even a rapidly moving structure such as the myocardium to be visualized with little motion blur. The rotation of the electron beam can be synchronized via ECG gating with the cardiac motion to produce images of the heart in various phases of the cardiac cycle; this technique is useful for functional imaging.[2]

Helical and electron beam CT scanners provide large numbers of thin, closely spaced slices, ideally suited to computer manipulation. Imaging workstations are actually specialized computers designed to manipulate cross-sectional image data. Workstations take successive cross-sectional imaging slices and create 3D matrices which may be manipulated easily. Thus, these workstations produce multiplanar

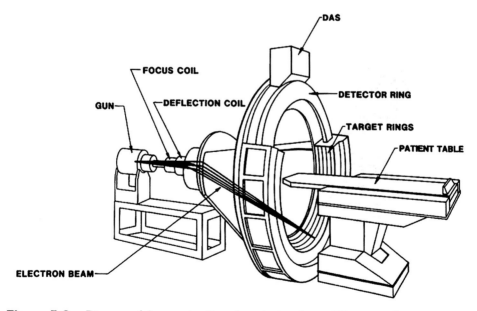

Figure 5.2. Diagram of the construction of an electron beam CT scanner. Large magnetic deflection coils sweep the beam of electrons around the tungsten target rings to produce x-rays which are then projected onto the patient table. A ring of detectors parallels the target rings and receives the x-rays after having passed through the patient. Reproduced with permission from Imatron Co.

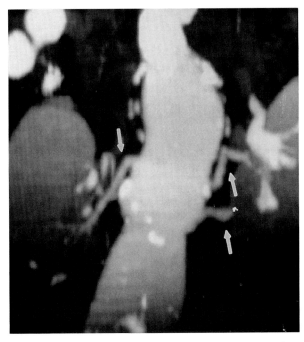

Figure 5.3.   Anterior view of a maximum intensity projection (MIP) of the abdominal aorta with a large upper abdominal aneurysm. Note the excellent visualization of the renal arteries (arrows) relative to the aneurysm.

reconstructions rapidly within any prescribed imaging plane. This application is especially useful in the thoracic aorta, where an imaging plane parallel to the entire course of the aorta, similar to that seen on a right posterior oblique (RPO) thoracic aortogram. Likewise, coronal reconstructions in the abdominal aorta are useful for visualization of the relationship of the renal arteries to aneurysms (Figure 5.3). If the original slices are sufficiently thin, smaller vessels, such as the renal or carotid arteries, may be visualized accurately.

Advanced workstations increase the intensity difference between contrast-enhanced blood and its surrounding structures to obtain arteriogram-like images referred to as maximum intensity projections (MIP). Through a series of mathematical manipulations, workstations construct 3D renderings of the luminal contour of major vessels with remarkable clarity. These surface shaded volume (SSV) renderings may be rotated to simulate viewing vessels at multiple angles (Figure 5.4). New computer techniques create data sets from the interior of major vessels; these vessels can then be viewed from a perspective similar to that seen with an endoscope. A virtual endoscopic inspection of the interior of a vessel is performed similar to bronchoscopy. The use of workstations to evaluate CT data sets is relatively new, but it will constitute a major tool in the use of CT scanning for evaluation of the cardiovascular system in the next few years[3] (Figure 5.5).

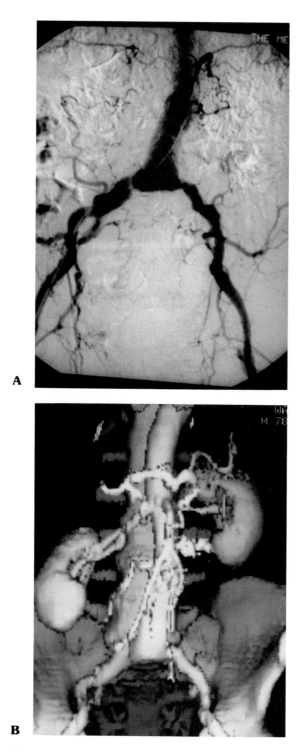

A

B

Figure 5.4. (A) Anterior view of the abdominal aorta from a digital subtraction arteriogram. There is aneurysmal change at the bifurcation with extensive atherosclerotic plaquing at the origin of the iliac. (B) Three-dimensional demonstration of the same abdominal aorta with surface shaped technique. Portions of the skeleton, branch vessels, and kidneys remain to demonstrate anatomic relationships.

(continued on next page)

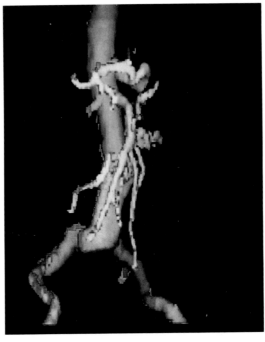

C

Figure 5.4. (C) The surface shaded model demonstrated in (B) has been further refined to leave only vascular structures. This has been rotated approximately 20° to a slightly oblique projection.

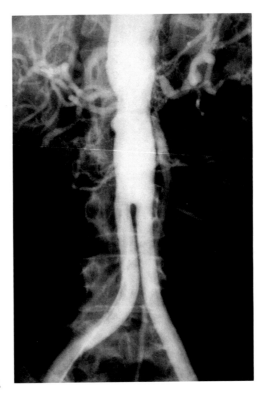

A

Figure 5.5. (A) Conventional contrast arteriogram of abdominal aortic bifurcation graft.

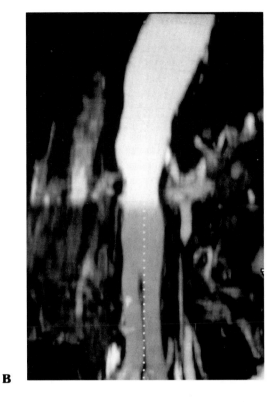

B

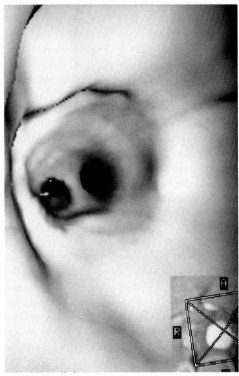

C

Figure 5.5. (B) Anterior MIP simulating arteriogram. This image was constructed from 60 individual helical CT scans acquired within a single 30-sec breath-hold. (C) Virtual endoscopic view of the interior of the aortic bifurcation graft created from the same data as (B).

INDICATIONS AND USES

Aorta and Branches

Noncontrast CT scans are adequate for the identification and evaluation of most aneurysms. Diameters are easily obtained and serial measurements are highly reproducible allowing accurate identification of interval aneurysm growth. Changes in the tissue planes surrounding the aorta are indicative of leaking or mycotic aneurysms. The addition of intravenous material and rapid helical CT scanning allows accurate determination of the relationship of aneurysms to major branch vessels, such as the renal arteries. If axial CT scans are reconstructed into sagittal and coronal projections, adequate detail is then available to plan surgical procedures.[4,5] Localized aortic ulcerations are likewise easily recognized on postcontrast CT scanning, and these may be differentiated from luminal irregularities caused by plaque and thrombus.[6]

Helical CT scanning with rapid infusion of intravenous contrast material allows the accurate identification and delineation of aortic dissections. The key findings are differential opacification of the two lumens and the actual visualization of the displaced intima (Figure 5.6). Secondary signs include thrombosed channels, displaced intimal calcifications, and aneurysmal dilatation. Multiplanar reconstructions visualize the actual contour of the aorta in a fashion exactly analogous to the standard three projections of the thoracic aorta and two projections of the abdominal aorta obtained through arteriography.[7,8] Decreased contrast enhancement identifies

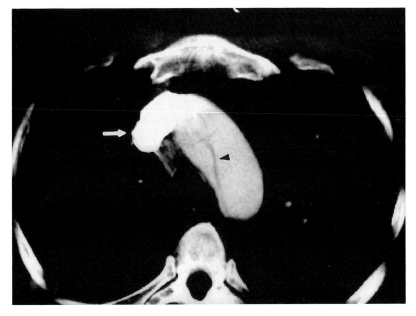

Figure 5.6.   Single slice from helical CT scan of the abdominal aorta at the level of the aortic arch. Dense contrast material is noted in the brachiocephalic vein as it merges with the superior vena cava (arrow). A clear intimal reflection (arrowhead) can be seen in the mid arch of the aorta. A complex type 1 dissection was present.

occlusion or involvement of major visceral branches. Intimal flaps may be visualized extending directly into these vessels. CT is unreliable in the evaluation of aortic insufficiency which often occurs with type A dissections. CT's sensitivity is competitive with MRI and transesophageal echocardiogram but is more widely available.

Traumatic interruption of the thoracic aorta is diagnosed both by the visualization of mediastinal hematoma and the subtle discontinuity of the aortic lumen on 3D reconstructions of the arch and thoracic aorta.[9] The exam time is typically less than 5 min; often this is a crucial consideration in dealing with complications of aneurysms or dissections. CT scanning under these conditions will supplant catheter angiography for the evaluation of the aorta.[10–12]

Very thin (1–3 mm) axial CT scans reconstruct into fine detail views of major branch vessels capable of delineating stenosis, occlusion, and aneurysm. This technique has been applied with success in the renal arteries, carotid arteries, and circle of Willis (Figures 5.7 and 5.8).

Pulmonary Artery

Major anomalies of the pulmonary arteries are identifiable on CT scans. Rapid scanning with intravenous contrast infusion allows evaluation of pulmonary artery diameters, stenoses, and anomalous connections. The involvement of the pulmonary arteries by a mediastinal tumor or by a tumor thrombus can be clearly delineated.

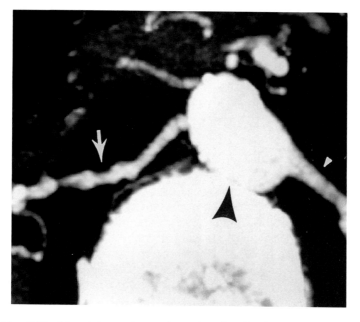

Figure 5.7. MIP of the abdominal aorta (arrowhead) and right renal artery (arrow) as seen from an inferior projection. Note the nodularity of the contour of the right renal artery, typical of fibromuscular hyperplasia. The left renal artery is smooth and regular (small arrowhead).

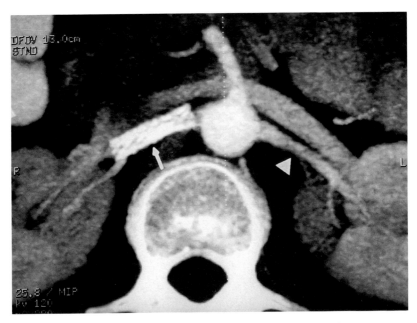

A

Figure 5.8. (A) Maximum intensity projection from helical CT scan focused on the renal arteries. Section actually consists of 18 1-mm-thick sections summated and intensified for visualization of the contrast material in the renal arteries. Note metallic stent which has been used to expand stenosis in the proximal right renal artery (*arrow*). The left renal artery (*arrowhead*) has a normal contour.

The rapid slice acquisition capabilities of electron beam CT scanners have proven to be reliable in the identification of major pulmonary emboli within the right and left pulmonary arteries and first order branches (Figure 5.9). It may be possible to identify pulmonary emboli reasonably well with helical CT scanning as well, although studies are incomplete at this time.[13–15] Nuclear medicine V-Q scans are considered more sensitive and pulmonary angiography remains the gold standard.

Vena Cava

Most anomalies of the vena cava are identifiable on standard CT scans. The use of intravenous contrast material allows the visualization of the involvement of vena cava by tumors and the extent of tumor thrombus spread along the course of the vena cava. Unfortunately, the identification of the involvement of the vena cava by tumor is not a reliable indicator of resectability; many intraluminal tumor thrombi are not solidly adherent to the wall of the vena cava. CT scans demonstrate vena caval occlusion reliably.[16]

Heart

Until the advent of electron beam CT scanning, cardiac visualization met with limited success due to motion artifact. With single slice scan times of 50 msec, freeze-

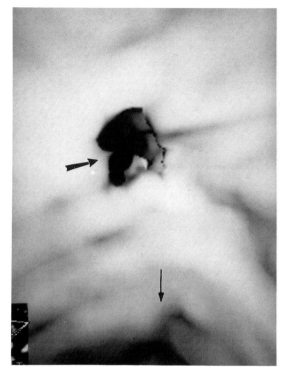

B

Figure 5.8. (B) Three-dimensional virtual endoscopy view of the orifice of the right renal artery as seen from the left wall of the abdominal aorta. Note the irregular contour at the orifice due to intimal ingrowth over the projections of the metallic stent (*arrow*). This projection was produced from the same data set as the image in (A). *Long arrow* points toward inferior abdominal aorta.

frame visualization of the heart is a reality. Noncontrast electron beam CT scanning of the heart has been extensively utilized in the visualization of calcium deposits within the coronary arteries (Figure 5.10). Numerous studies establish a significant correlation between the volume of calcium deposited within the coronary arteries as calculated from thin sectioned CT scans and the likelihood of atherosclerotic coronary artery disease. These measurements are rapid, reproducible and highly indicative of the state of atherosclerosis within the coronary arteries. Several studies have established the relationship of coronary artery calcium quantity to positive findings on coronary angiography. The role of this technique in the evaluation and screening of patients for atherosclerotic coronary artery disease is evolving.[17–19]

One of the most attractive potential roles of cardiac ultrafast CT imaging may be in the early detection of coronary atherosclerosis among asymptomatic patients who have risk factors for development of coronary artery disease. Several studies have demonstrated that patients without coronary calcification have a very low likelihood of significant (≥50%) coronary artery stenosis, whereas the extent and severity of coronary artery disease clearly correlates with the number of coronary artery calcifications that are observed.

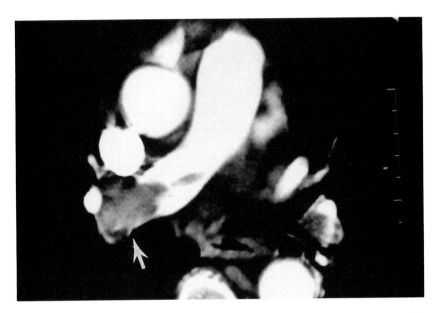

Figure 5.9. Single slice from helical CT scan through the right pulmonary artery after the administration of intravenous contrast material. Note the defect (*arrow*) occluding the artery, representing large adherent thrombus.

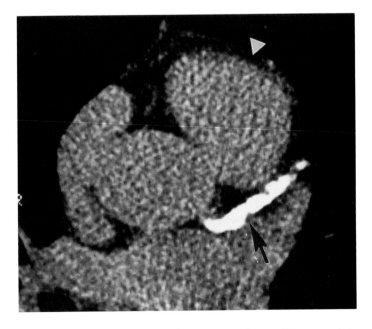

Figure 5.10. Thin section slice (3 mm) from electron beam CT scan of the origin and proximal course of the left anterior descending artery (*arrow*). There is extensive calcification indicative of a high degree of atherosclerotic disease. *Arrowhead* identifies pulmonary artery outflow tract.

Patients with minimal or no coronary artery calcification might therefore only require appropriate risk factor modification without any further cardiac evaluation. On the other hand, patients with more extensive (moderate/severe) calcification might best be further evaluated with myocardial perfusion imaging to determine whether significant flow-limiting coronary stenoses are present. Coronary angiography would be performed only in this latter group of patients. Published reports indicate that the majority of asymptomatic patients screened with ultrafast CT imaging have indeed only mild or no coronary calcification, which thereby allows rapid screening of a large number of patients at risk with relatively few undergoing invasive cardiac procedures. Recent trials have also demonstrated that patients without coronary artery calcification have an excellent prognosis up to 5 yr after the initial scan, reinforcing the concept that these patients who represent a sizable percentage of those with risk factors for coronary artery disease need only medical management and aggressive risk factor modification. The role of ultrafast CT imaging in patients with angina and known coronary artery disease would at this time seem moot since the severity and location of coronary stenosis cannot be determined from the location of coronary artery calcium. Further study is necessary to better define the niche that ultrafast CT imaging will ultimately occupy in the diagnosis and evaluation of patients with coronary artery disease.

Electron beam CT scanning during the infusion of bolus intravenous contrast material allows visualization of the coronary arteries with sufficient clarity to diagnose aneurysms and major anomalies. Several studies have demonstrated the usefulness of this technique in evaluating the patency of coronary artery bypass grafts; 3D workstation techniques simulate actual surface reconstructions of bypass grafts. Dynamic flow studies are performed during a single pass of iodinated contrast. Abnormal bypass grafts are diagnosed from intensity curves plotted from regions of interest taken over the ascending aorta and bypass grafts. Significant challenges remain in this area. Preliminary results indicate a role for computed tomography in the evaluation of the native coronary arteries within the near future.[20,21]

Contrast infusion studies may be used to visualize tumor or thrombus within the cardiac chambers (Figure 5.11). Dynamic studies at multiple levels during multiple phases of the cardiac cycle allow evaluation of regional wall motion, ejection fraction, and other parameters of cardiac dynamics.[2,22]

ADVANTAGES AND DISADVANTAGES

CT scanners are not portable devices; their use is limited to patients sufficiently stable to allow transport to the site of the CT scanner. Examinations requiring iodinated contrast material entail the risk of allergic reactions, as with other techniques, but this has been significantly reduced in recent years with the advent of nonionic contrast material and pharmacologic prophylaxis.

The speed of helical and electron beam CT scanners allows for the rapid performance of most examinations. Except for the need of peripheral intravenous access, CT examinations are almost entirely noninvasive. CT techniques examine many aspects of the cardiovascular system with considerable reduction in the risk of procedure-related complications. The cost of a CT scan is approximately one-third

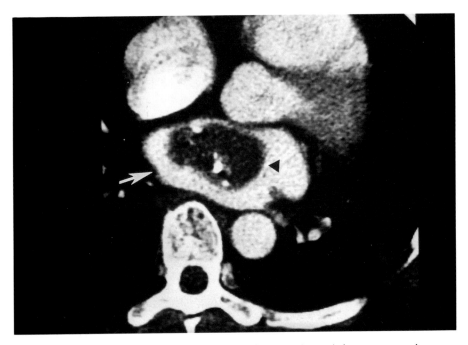

Figure 5.11.   Electron beam CT scan of the left atrium (*arrow*) demonstrating large myxomatous tumor (*arrowhead*) with punctate calcifications.

that of traditional angiographic procedures of the major vessels; yet, it provides equivalent information. New data predictive of atherosclerotic coronary artery disease is available with coronary artery calcium scans at a cost competitive with exercise ECG.[23]

FUTURE ADVANCEMENT

The evolution of helical and electron beam CT scanning since 1990 has been remarkable. The rapidity with which new facets of these techniques have been developed indicates that there are many new applications just over the horizon. Improvements in the operating software of computerized workstations will allow more rapid construction of 3D images of the vessels, as well as produce enhanced contrast within flat representations of the vessels, such as maximum intensity projections. It is possible to inspect visually the lumina of vessels with CT virtual endoscopy, a reality awaiting sufficient clinical trials to validate its accuracy. Functional assessment of the myocardium, as well as other organs, such as the kidney, will become more widespread as scanning techniques allow the rapid acquisition of multiple images within the short time period required for perfusion of an organ.[24]

SUMMARY

Computed tomography within the cardiovascular system has developed rapidly since the introduction of new CT scanners. These devices have allowed a shift of utilization away from more traditional and invasive imaging modalities, such as angiography. The future applications of computed tomography of the cardiovascular system may well begin to rival current applications of nuclear medicine techniques.

REFERENCES

1. Brink JA: Technical aspects of helical (spiral) CT. *Radiol Clin North Am* 33:825–841, 1995.
2. McCollough CH, Morin RL: The technical design and performance of ultrafast computed tomography. *Radiol Clin North Am* 32:521–536, 1994.
3. Ehricke HH, Grynert T, Buck T, et al: Medical workstations for applied imaging and graphics research. *Comput Med Imag Graph* 18:403, 1994.
4. Van Hoe L, Baert AL, Gryspeerdt S, et al: Supra- and juxtarenal aneurysms of the abdominal aorta: preoperative assessment with thin-section spiral CT. *Radiology* 198:443–448, 1996.
5. Zeman RK, Silverman PM, Berman PM, et al: Abdominal aortic aneurysms: evaluation with variable-collimation helical CT and overlapping reconstruction. *Radiology* 193:555–560, 1994.
6. Harris JA, Bis KG, Glover JL, et al: Penetrating atherosclerotic ulcers of the aorta. *J Vasc Surg* 19:90–99, 1994.
7. Zeman RK, Berman PM, Silverman PM, et al: Diagnosis of aortic dissection: value of helical CT with multiplanar reformation and three-dimensional rendering. *Am J Radiol* 164:1375–1380, 1995.
8. Cigarroa JE, Isselbacher EM, DeSanctis RW, et al: Medical progress. Diagnostic imaging in the evaluation of suspected aortic dissection: old standards and new directions. *N Engl J Med* 328:35–43, 1993.
9. Gavant ML, Menke PG, Fabian T, et al: Blunt traumatic aortic rupture: detection with helical CT of the chest. *Radiology* 197:125–133, 1995.
10. Platt JF, Ellis JH, Korobkin M, et al: Potential renal donors: comparison of conventional imaging with helical CT. *Radiology* 198:419–423, 1996.
11. Rubin GD, Alfrey EJ, Dake MD, et al: Assessment of living renal donors with spiral CT. *Radiology* 195:457–462, 1995.
12. Alberico RA, Patel M, Casey S, et al: Evaluation of the circle of Willis with three-dimensional CT angiography in patients with suspected intracranial aneurysms. *Am J Neuroradiol* 16:1571–1578, 1995.
13. Touliopoulos P, Costello P: Helical (spiral) CT of the thorax. *Radiol Clin North Am* 33:843–861, 1995.
14. Remy J, Remy-Jardin M, Giraud F, et al: Angioarchitecture of pulmonary arteriovenous malformations; clinical utility of three-dimensional helical CT. *Radiology* 191:657–664, 1994.

15. Goodman LR, Curtin JJ, Mewissen MW, et al: Detection of pulmonary embolism in patients with unresolved clinical and scintigraphic diagnosis: helical CT versus angiography. *Am J Radiol* 164:1369–1374, 1995.

16. Ibukuro K, Charnsangavej C, Chasen MH, et al: Helical CT angiography with multiplanar reformation: techniques and clinical applications. *RadioGraphics* 15:671–682, 1995.

17. Agatston AS, Janowitz WR, Hildner FJ, et al: Quantification of coronary artery calcium using ultrafast computed tomography. *J Am Coll Cardiol* 15:827–832, 1990.

18. Budoff MJ, Georgiou D, Brody A, et al: Ultrafast computed tomography as a diagnostic modality in the detection of coronary artery disease: a multicenter study. *Circulation* 93:898–904, 1996.

19. Mautner GC, Mautner SL, Froehlich J, et al: Coronary artery calcification: assessment with electron beam CT and histomorphometric correlation. *Radiology* 192:619–623, 1994.

20. Tello R, Costello P, Ecker C, et al: Spiral CT evaluation of coronary artery bypass graft patency. *J Comput Assist Tomogr* 17:253–259, 1993.

21. Moshage WEL, Achenbach S, Seese B, et al: Coronary artery stenoses: three-dimensional imaging with electrocardiographically triggered, contrast agent–enhanced, electron-beam CT. *Radiology* 196:707–714, 1995.

22. Thompson BH, Stanford W: Evaluation of cardiac function with ultrafast computed tomography. *Radiol Clin North Am* 32:537–551, 1994.

23. Bluemke DA, Chambers TP: Spiral CT angiography: an alternative to conventional angiography. *Radiology* 195:317–319, 1995.

24. Rubin GD, Dake MD, Semba CP: Current status of three-dimensional spiral CT scanning for imaging the vasculature. *Radiol Clin North Am* 33:51–70, 1995.

— Section 2 —
SEMI-INVASIVE DIAGNOSTIC PROCEDURES

—6—

Transesophageal Echocardiography

William A. Zoghbi, M.D.

Over the past two decades, major advances have occurred in the field of echocardiography including high-resolution imaging, the refinement of Doppler technology, and digital acquisition of ultrasound images. Among these innovations, transesophageal echocardiography (TEE) clearly represents a major breakthrough which has recently incorporated all the technological advances of echocardiography and currently provides a powerful diagnostic tool in the evaluation of the cardiac patient. While transthoracic echocardiography remains the most commonly used ultrasound modality and offers several advantages by being totally noninvasive and providing multiple windows for imaging and Doppler interrogation, it has several limitations due to the acoustic attenuation from the thorax, valve calcifications, and prosthetic valves. With the proximity of the esophagus to the posterior cardiac structures and the aorta, TEE obviates several of these limitations and provides a complementary imaging technique to that of transthoracic echocardiography. Furthermore, high-frequency transducers can be used which provide increased resolution of ultrasound images. This chapter will briefly discuss the technique of TEE and emphasizes the indications of this modality in the evaluation of the cardiac patient.

DESCRIPTION OF THE TECHNIQUE

With TEE, the ultrasound transducer is located at a tip of a scope that is advanced through the oropharynx into the esophagus and stomach. Because of the proximity of the heart and aorta to the esophagus and the stomach, imaging of these cardio-

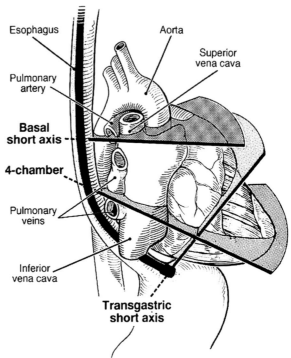

Figure 6.1. Schematic representation of transesophageal echocardiography showing the relation of the TEE probe in the esophagus and stomach to the cardiovascular structures. The plane of imaging shown is that of the horizontal plane. In biplane probes, a longitudinal plane orthogonal to the one shown is also available. In multiplane TEE probes, the imaging plane can be rotated in 180° angulation. In addition, the tip of the probe can be remotely manipulated in different directions.

vascular structures can be easily performed (Figure 6.1). The imaging plane emanates in a perpendicular fashion to the shaft of the transducer and can be advanced and rotated sideways by advancing and rotating the probe. Furthermore, the tip of the probe can be manipulated in several directions (antiflexion, retroflexion, and sideflexion) to interrogate and further define the structures imaged. A schematic description of visualization of the cardiac structures with TEE is shown in Figure 6.1. In addition to the imaging plane depicted, new technology has allowed imaging in orthogonal planes (biplane) and rotating the image 180° (multiplane), thus allowing further refinement in imaging and flow interrogation.

DEVELOPMENTAL PERSPECTIVES

Initial attempts at transesophageal echocardiography date back to 1976 when Frazin et al.[1] described their initial experience with a single crystal transducer attached to a coaxial cable passed through the esophagus which allowed M mode cardiac imaging. Subsequently, multicrystal ultrasound transducers were attached to modified gastroscopes; cross-sectional echocardiography was performed with mechanical scanning. Significant advancement came with incorporation of phased-array transducers,[2] initially to modified gastroscopes and more recently to probes specifically designed for TEE. Color flow Doppler, pulsed, and continuous wave Doppler were incorporated. Concomitant with these developments, echocardiographic planes evolved from a monoplane, allowing imaging in the horizontal plane only (Figure 6.1) to biplane imaging (in two orthogonal planes).[3–5] The longitudinal plane is particularly helpful in imaging the superior vena cava, interatrial septum, ascending aorta, the atrial appendages, and the left ventricle. In 1991, multiplane imaging was introduced and allowed steering the imaging plane in incremental rotations up to 180°, adding further refinement to imaging and flow interrogation.[6,7] Currently, biplane and multiplane TEE technologies are widely available and are used interchangeably in most echocardiography laboratories.

TECHNICAL CONSIDERATIONS

The TEE procedure can be performed in the echocardiography laboratory for outpatients or hospitalized individuals, in the operating room or any other location, provided that the necessary equipment is available. The patient must refrain from oral intake of solids or liquids for at least 4 hr prior to the examination. Pertinent history should be elicited, particularly with the emphasis on symptoms or pathology relating to the gastrointestinal tract such as dysphasia, gastroesophageal disorders, recent upper gastrointestinal surgical procedure as well as drug allergies. Dentures or oral prosthesis must be removed before the examination. An intravenous access is obtained in all patients.

After the administration of local anesthesia to the oropharynx, the study is performed with the patient in the left lateral decubitus position, to minimize the risk of aspiration. Depending on the clinical condition, other positions are possible (right lateral, prone, or sitting position). Further details on the technical aspects of introduction of the TEE probe, examination, and images obtained have been previously described and are beyond the scope of this chapter.[3,4,7] Intravenous sedation and analgesics are administered as needed to ensure comfort and cooperation during the study. Whether antibiotic prophylaxis against endocarditis should be administered has not been resolved. Recent studies have shown that bacteremia is rarely associated with TEE.[8,9] We and others[10] do not recommend prophylaxis against endocarditis before the procedure and are not aware of any cases with endocarditis complicating several thousands of transesophageal echocardiograms performed in these institutions. Others have recommended endocarditis prophylaxis in patients with prosthetic valves, poor dentition, or previous infective endocarditis.[11]

Since TEE is an invasive procedure, it should not be used routinely and should be performed only by trained physicians, specialized in the procedure. Recommendations for the performance and maintenance of skills of TEE have been recently published by the American Society of Echocardiography.[12] Various imaging planes to interrogate cardiac structures and flows can be obtained by several maneuvers of the probe shaft itself (advancement, rotation, flexion or retroflexion of the tip, side flexion) as well as switching between horizontal and longitudinal planes or those in between with multiplane imaging.[3,4,7,13] Similar to any other diagnostic modality, it is imperative to have a methodical approach during the performance of a transesophageal echocardiogram to obtain all possible information from the study. It is our practice once the transesophageal probe is in place to first address the clinical question. This is performed in case the examination has to be interrupted prematurely. Once this is defined, we proceed with all regular views, from the transesophageal level to the transgastric views and ending with imaging of the aorta. Regardless of the indication of the study, a comprehensive examination of all the regions of the heart and the great vessels in our experience yields, not infrequently (7%), incidental yet important cardiovascular findings, not suspected clinically.

INDICATIONS AND USES

Currently, transesophageal echocardiography complements the transthoracic approach in a subset of patients. In general, the transthoracic examination is performed first, and if the clinical question cannot be answered, the transesophageal echocardiogram is recommended. In our experience as well as others,[10,14] TEE is performed in approximately 5% to 8% of patients undergoing surface echocardiograms. Indications for transesophageal echocardiography have grown rapidly and are summarized in Table 6.1. The distribution of these indications in a particular laboratory varies predominantly depending on the patient population referred and practice patterns. The most common indications, excluding the operating room setting, have been evaluation of sources of emboli, suspected endocarditis, and assessment of prosthetic valve function.

Sources of Embolism

Transthoracic echocardiography has long been used for the evaluation of patients with possible cardiac sources of emboli. Recent data, however, reveals that several potential sources for embolism can frequently be missed with this technique.[15–17] This is predominantly due to the poor resolution of echocardiographic images in the cardiac base, left atrial appendage, and aorta. In studies that have compared transesophageal with transthoracic echocardiography, TEE has clearly shown superiority in identifying potential sources of embolus such as left atrial appendate thrombi, left

TABLE 6.1.   General Indications for Transesophageal Echocardiography

Cardiac sources of emboli
Suspected prosthetic valve dysfunction
Evaluation of cardiac masses and tumors
Suspected endocarditis
Assessment of valvular morphology and regurgitation
The critically ill patient with possible cardiac etiology
Diseases of the aorta
Congenital heart disease
Technically difficult transthoracic echocardiogram
Guidance during interventional procedures
Planning and assessment of results of cardiac surgery
Cardiac monitoring during high-risk surgical procedures

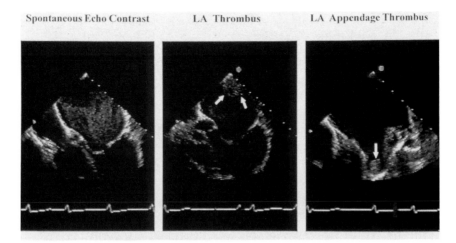

Figure 6.2. Example of a patient with mitral stenosis in whom the TEE was performed to exclude thrombus formation prior to balloon valvuloplasty. Spontaneous echo contrast in the left atrium and thrombus formation in the left atrium (two arrows) and in left atrial appendage (arrow) are shown.

atrial thrombi, vegetations on native or prosthetic valves, interatrial aneurysms, and patent foramen ovale.[15,17,18] Spontaneous echo contrast, a phenomenon associated with slow blood flow, is more frequently identified with TEE, and has been associated with increased risk for thromboembolic events.[19,20] Spontaneous echo contrast is most often seen in the left atrium in patients with mitral stenosis, mitral prosthetic valves, or atrial fibrillation (Figure 6.2).

Recently, with the advent of TEE, it has been more clearly realized that the aorta can be a significant potential source of cerebral and peripheral embolization. Patients with complex atheromas in the aorta, particularly those associated with mobile "aortic debris" found recently to be thrombus, have a high likelihood for embolization[21] (Figure 6.3). As to left ventricular thrombi, the transthoracic and transesophageal approaches are comparable in the detection of this lesion in view of the fact that left ventricular thrombi complicating previous myocardial infarction or cardiomyopathy are usually located in the cardiac apex. TEE in these situations is reserved for technically difficult or suspicious cases.

While the yield of TEE is higher in detecting potential sources of embolism, proving causality of the ultrasound findings in the embolic episode may be difficult. The presence of thrombi and/or masses provides as close a direct evidence as possible for an embolic source. However, the presence of only possible causes such as patent foramen ovale or interatrial aneurysms provides less strong evidence. The ultimate question remains: Should TEE be performed routinely in a patient with a possible embolic stroke or a peripheral vascular event? Although these recommendations are still being refined, transthoracic echocardiography is still currently most often obtained. If a source is identified, TEE is not routinely performed. At Baylor College Of Medicine, TEE is performed in patients with unexplained embolic event, more often in younger and middle-aged individuals and particularly if the results of the TEE would alter management. In patients who will be receiving anticoagulation, irrespective of TEE findings (e.g., atrial fibrillation), this procedure would not be recommended.

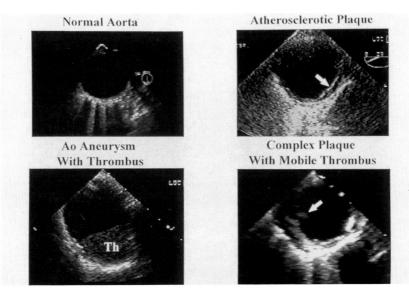

Figure 6.3. Cross-section of the aorta showing a normal aorta in short axis and various pathologies that could be visualized with transesophageal echocardiography. The atherosclerotic plaque and mobile thrombus are depicted by arrow; Th = Thrombus.

The role of TEE prior to electrical cardioversion for atrial fibrillation is being investigated.[18,22] Although intuitively a negative TEE for atrial thrombi would suggest a safe cardioversion, recent data have shown that embolic phenomena after cardioversion can occur with a negative TEE if patients are not appropriately anticoagulated.[23] This is most likely related to the phenomenon of atrial stunning after cardioversion.[24,25] Thus, anticoagulation so far is necessary at the time of cardioversion and for approximately 1 month afterwards.[18] However, TEE has been shown to decrease the need for prolonged anticoagulation prior to cardioversion.[18] Although generalization of the use of TEE to all patients with atrial fibrillation is premature and is currently under study, it can be used in hospitalized patients, in those with tenuous hemodynamic status, and in patients with contraindication to anticoagulation.

Endocarditis and Its Cardiac Complications

Valvular vegetations are the hallmark of infective endocarditis. Although the diagnosis of this entity continues to depend on bedside evaluation and bacteriologic confirmation, echocardiography has assumed a pivotal role in both diagnosis and management of patients with endocarditis. With current improvements in instrumentation and the availability of TEE, the technique provides detection of vegetations, evaluation of location, extent and size of vegetations, recognition of perivalvular complications from the infection such as valve destruction, root abscess, and fistula formation. Importantly, echocardiography also provides accurate evaluation of the severity of valvular regurgitation and the functional status of the left ventricle.

Transthoracic echocardiography has been reported to be between 60–80% sensitive for the detection of vegetations with a high specificity, usually over 90.[26–28]

Detection of vegetations is dependent on its size, location, and the presence of prosthetic valve. The most difficult vegetations to recognize are those present in a prosthetic valve. The high ultrasound reflections from the valve itself make it often impossible to recognize the presence of any mass attached to the valve. Sometimes, if these vegetations are large enough or if attached to a porcine prosthesis or on the ventricular side of the prosthesis, they can be recognized with routine transthoracic examination. Detection of prosthetic valve vegetation is perhaps one of the greatest contributions of TEE.

TEE has significantly improved the detection of valvular vegetations and evaluation of complications of endocarditis. Several recent studies have compared transthoracic echocardiography with TEE in the detection of infective endocarditis.[26-28] In these studies, TEE has proven to be consistently superior to transthoracic imaging in detection of vegetations and complications, particularly in prosthetic valves. Overall, in native valve endocarditis, TEE is >95% sensitive for detection of vegetation. False-negative results may result from very small vegetations, leaflet perforation without an obvious vegetation. In prosthetic valves, TEE is exceedingly superior to transthoracic echo in the detection of vegetations (Figure 6.4). In native valve endocarditis, a normal TEE (valve structure and function) virtually excludes endocarditis.[28] In our experience, a negative TEE in patients referred for evaluation of endocarditis prompted more aggressive search and ultimate finding of other sources of infection and was associated with a lower duration of antibiotic administration and hospitalization.[28] In prosthetic valves, however, although a negative TEE examination decreases significantly the likelihood of endocarditis, it does not exclude it.[28] In certain situations, differentiation between active endocarditis from other types of valvular masses may be difficult, particularly with transthoracic imaging and

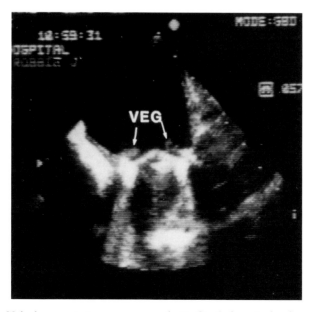

Figure 6.4. Valvular vegetations on a prosthetic St. Jude mitral valve on the left atrial side, shown by arrows. Despite adequate surface echocardiography, vegetations could not be seen.

even with TEE. These include old healed or calcified vegetations, areas of focal valvular calcification or sclerosis, papillomas, and myxomatous changes in a mitral valve. Integration of clinical, laboratory, and ultrasound findings is specially needed in these situations to direct patient management.

The main clinical complications of endocarditis include embolization, development of heart failure secondary to valvular insufficiency or myocardial dysfunction, intractable infection resistant to antibiotic therapy, and ultimately death. The severity of valve involvement and degree of regurgitation, the presence of perivalvular abscesses, the type of valve infected (native versus prosthetic; right-sided versus left-sided), and the size of the vegetations are important factors that influence the ultimate clinical course. In recent studies, vegetations >10 mm in size were associated with a higher risk for embolization.[26] There has been no significant correlation between the size of vegetation and the infective organism or the type of valve infected. Likewise, the size of vegetation has related less well with other complications of endocarditis. On the other hand, the presence of significant valvular regurgitation, perivalvular abscesses, or fistulae are all associated with a greater need for early surgery and, in some studies, with a higher mortality.

Although detection of a perivalvular abscess is possible with transthoracic examination, it is infrequent, particularly in the presence of a prosthetic valve. TEE has been shown to be more accurate in the recognition of abscess formation.[29–31] In aortic valve endocarditis, a particular predilection to involvement of the aortic–mitral intervalvular fibrosa has been demonstrated, with abscess and pseudoaneurysm formation.[30,31] This entity is usually missed by transthoracic echocardiography and is best visualized with TEE. A recent study from our institution revealed that TEE is even superior to aortography in diagnosing this complication.[31] Opacification of the pseudoaneurysm, which communicates with the left ventricle, does not occur with an injection of contrast in the aortic root unless concomitant aortic insufficiency is present (Figure 6.5).

Conventional transthoracic examination is accurate for the evaluation of the severity of native valvular regurgitation. On the other hand, regurgitation associated with prosthetic valves, as discussed later in this chapter, can be more difficult to evaluate particularly in the mitral position, due to the increased reflections from the prosthesis and decreasing the intensity of the Doppler ultrasound signal reaching the left atrium. TEE provides a highly sensitive and accurate technique for detection of prosthetic valve regurgitation and evaluation of the site of regurgitation. An important cause of "mitral regurgitation" in patients with prosthetic aortic valve endocarditis is a communication between the left ventricular outflow and the left atrium through a fistula (Figure 6.6) or through an aortic root abscess that ruptures into the left atrium.[31,32]

In summary, echocardiography is currently a highly valuable technique in patients with suspected or known infective endocarditis. Transthoracic examination should be performed in every patient suspected of having native valvular disease and the threshold for TEE should be fairly low, particularly if the transthoracic examination fails to reveal findings of endocarditis and the clinical picture is highly suggestive of this entity. Suggested indications of TEE in patients with suspected native valve endocarditis based on the transthoracic echo findings are listed in Table 6.2. Patients with a prosthetic valve suspected of having endocarditis, on the other hand should routinely undergo a TEE examination because of its vast superiority over

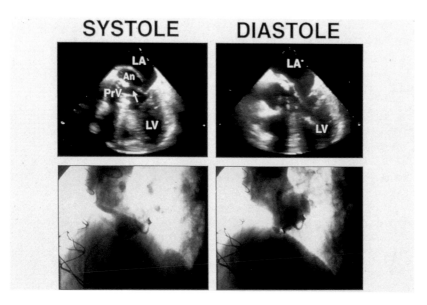

Figure 6.5. Patient with a pseudoaneurysm of the mitral-aortic intervalvular fibrosa complicating prosthetic aortic valve endocarditis showing pulsatility of the pseudoaneurysm (an) because of its communication with the left ventricle only. Aortic root injection of contrast does not visualize this abnormality. The arrow points to the site of communication of the pseudoaneurysm to the left ventricular outflow tract. An = pseudoaneurysm; LA = Left atrium; LV = left ventricle; PrV = prosthetic aortic valve. Reproduced with permission from the American College Of Cardiology from Ref. 31.

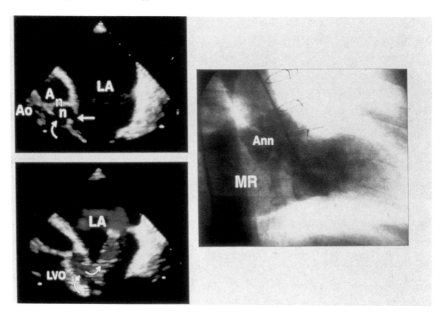

Figure 6.6. Demonstration of a ruptured abscess in the aortic-mitral intervalvular fibrosa complicating endocarditis. The pseudoaneurysm (Ann) acts as a conduit between the left ventricle (LV) and atrium (LA) and "mitral regurgitation" occurs through this communication. Left ventricular angiography demonstrates the mitral regurgitation (MR) but does not elucidate its mechanism. The curved arrow shows entry site from left ventricular outflow and straight arrow shows rupture site of the pseudoaneurysm into the left atrium. AO = aorta; LVO = left ventricular outflow tract. Reproduced with permission from the American College Of Cardiology from Ref. 31.

TABLE 6.2. Indications of TEE in Native Valve Endocarditis

Transthoracic echo findings:
  No definite vegetation seen:
    Nondiagnostic study (technically difficult, suspicious)
    Abormal valve structure and/or function
    Critically ill patients, despite adequate negative 2D echo
    Normal 2D echo/Doppler of adequate quality, in cases with high probability
  Definite vegetation seen:
    Failure of antibiotic therapy
    Evaluation of complications (abscess, fistula, rupture)
    Assessment of concomitant regurgitation (mechanism, severity)
    Preoperative evaluation

---

transthoracic approach in detection of vegetations, valvular regurgitation, and perivalvular abscesses. In the absence of coronary artery disease, the timing and planning of surgical interventions can be performed accurately with the information provided by echocardiography. In these patients, a TEE examination is indicated in all patients to define the extent of complications that need to be addressed surgically.

Prosthetic Valve Dysfunction

Prosthetic Valve Regurgitation

Regurgitation of prosthetic valves may arise from transvalvular or paravalvular leaks. With transthoracic echocardiography, the sensitivity and accuracy of Doppler techniques in the detection of prosthetic valve regurgitation depend largely on the position of the valve (e.g., aortic versus mitral). While transthoracic Doppler is very sensitive and accurate for the evaluation of aortic prosthetic valve regurgitation, it is quite limited in mitral prosthetic regurgitation, particularly if the prosthesis is a mechanical valve.[33,34] These problems arise from masking of the ultrasound signal behind the prosthetic valve, therefore hindering imaging as well as Doppler evaluation. TEE clearly represents a major advance in the evaluation of prosthetic valve regurgitation, particularly in the mitral position. In addition, TEE frequently allows for the distinction of the site of regurgitation, i.e., paravalvular versus transvalvular (Figure 6.7). In patients with biologic valves, TEE provides excellent image resolution of the valve leaflets allowing for accurate diagnosis of the mechanism of regurgitation. Criteria for evaluation of severity of prosthetic mitral valve regurgitation include assessment of the behavior of the regurgitant jet in the left atrium, the proximal acceleration and width of the jet, the degree of swirling within the atrium, and the presence and severity of retrograde regurgitant flow into the pulmonary veins. Several studies have demonstrated that this approach is considerably more accurate in prosthetic mitral valves than estimates obtained with the transthoracic approach.[33,34]

    On the other hand, for prosthetic aortic valves, the transthoracic approach often provides enough clues to distinguish mild from severe regurgitation, particularly when the appearance of the regurgitant jet by color is integrated with informa-

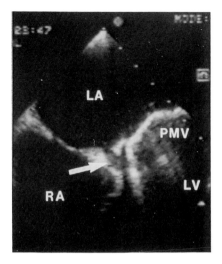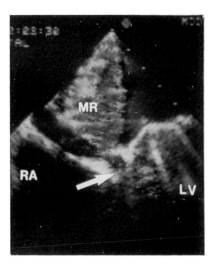

Figure 6.7. TEE showing severe mitral regurgitation occurring from a paravalvular leak in a prosthetic St. Jude Medical valve in the mitral position. The site of medial dehiscence is shown by arrow. This regurgitation was completely missed by surface echocardiography because of shadowing of the prosthesis from that view. The arrows point to the area of dehiscence. LA = left atrium; LV = left ventricle; MR = mitral regurgitation; PMV = prosthetic mitral valve; RA = right atrium.

tion from pressure half-time of the regurgitant jet by CW Doppler and with the degree of retrograde diastolic flow in the descending thoracic aorta.[35] TEE is usually reserved for technically difficult cases, to better define the mechanism of regurgitation and/or to assess the aortic root for associated pathology.[33,36] As discussed earlier, in patients with prosthetic valve endocarditis, aortic or mitral, TEE has become the diagnostic technique of choice for detection of vegetations as well as perivalvular regurgitation, annular abscesses, and fistula formation. Before the availability of TEE, many of these important pathologic conditions were missed by conventional transthoracic examination.

Prosthetic Valve Obstruction

The hemodynamic assessment of prosthetic valve function and diagnosis of prosthetic valve obstruction are well evaluated with transthoracic echocardiography, particularly with the use of pulsed and continuous wave Doppler. Measurements of jet velocity, mean gradients, and estimates of valve areas by Doppler result in accurate detection of significant prosthetic valve obstruction. Evaluation of prosthetic mitral valves includes determination of mean gradient, valve area by pressure half-time, and, in special cases, valve area by the continuity equation.[37,38] As to the aortic valve, function is evaluated with the determination of maximal and mean gradients, effective valve areas by the continuity equation as well as the Doppler velocity index (ratio of peak velocity by pulsed Doppler in the LV outflow, to the peak velocity through the prosthesis by CW Doppler).[37,39] Normal values for various valves and sizes have been reported.[37–39] For decisions in individual patients, the availability of a baseline Doppler evaluation of the prosthetic valve following valve replacement is always desirable for comparison.

Thus, in the vast majority of individuals, transthoracic Doppler examination is still the cornerstone for assessment of obstruction of a prosthetic valve. This results from the fact that the transthoracic approach allows multiple windows for Doppler interrogation of the stenotic jets, which are frequently eccentric. Furthermore, this approach allows evaluation of all the valves in question. Its limitations, however, are in the lower imaging resolution to define the *etiology* of the obstruction, particularly in mechanical valves. The obstruction can be due to thrombus, pannus formation, or mechanical dysfunction of the disk or poppet (Figure 6.8). Table 6.3 lists suggested indications for TEE in patients with suspected prosthetic valve obstruction. Accurate diagnosis of thrombus formation in a prosthetic valve may be important when thrombolytic therapy is considered as an alternative to surgery.[40–42] Transesophageal echocardiography allows the detection of thrombi adherent to a prosthetic valve, particularly in the mitral position since the majority of the thrombi are on the atrial side of the valve where image resolution is optimized. Pannus formation, on the other hand, may be at times difficult to visualize and the valve may appear relatively normal even though by continuous wave Doppler there is definite evidence of obstruction. Mechanical failure, on the other hand, can be frequently recognized by evaluating the motion of the disk.

Native Valve Disease

Valve Regurgitation

Transthoracic echocardiography remains the primary diagnostic tool for the evaluation of native valvular heart disease. A variety of parameters have been used for the assessment of valvular regurgitation and have been discussed in Chapter 1, including information from ventricular size and function, pulsed, and continuous wave Doppler as well as color flow imaging. Since each of these parameters may have some limitations, an optimum assessment of valvular regurgitation requires an integrated approach of several of these parameters. If the transthoracic approach is not diagnostic or offers only clues as to the severity of the regurgitant lesion, TEE is generally indicated to further define its severity and etiology.

Similar to prosthetic valves, evaluation of native aortic insufficiency can be performed in the majority of cases with the transthoracic approach. Although there are more limitations to the evaluation of mitral regurgitation, assessment of this lesion and its etiology in native valves can be performed in the majority of cases from the transthoracic approach. The most common situations where transthoracic color flow assessment can be misleading in the assessment of mitral regurgitation are: (1) the presence of the eccentric jets such as those seen with a flail mitral valve, where jet area significantly underestimates severity; (2) the presence of intense calcification of the mitral valve or annulus, which limits the ultrasound signal reaching the left atrium and may therefore produce underestimation of the severity of regurgitation; (3) in the presence of critically ill patients or those with tachycardia where the frame rate of the system may limit appreciation of the extent of the regurgitant jet in the left atrium.

In these cases, TEE may be extremely valuable for the assessment of the severity of regurgitation and delineation of its etiology.[43–45] The extension of the regurgitant jet into the left atrium can be very well seen and, in addition, one can assess

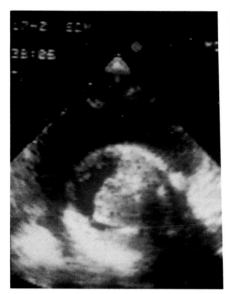 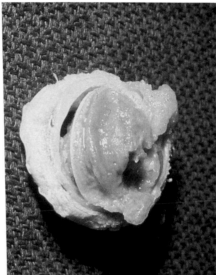

Figure 6.8. TEE examination in a patient presenting with shock and a nondiagnostic transthoracic exam. Obstruction and thrombus formation in the Bjork-Shiley prosthetic mitral valve is seen with a small area of flow. The pathologic correlate at surgery in this patient is shown.

the presence of retrograde regurgitant flow into the pulmonary veins, which indicates significant regurgitation.

Valve Stenosis

The severity of valvular stenosis can be assessed in the vast majority of cases with the transthoracic approach: virtually all cases of mitral, pulmonic, and tricuspid stenoses, and the majority of aortic stenosis (>95%). The methods involved have been described earlier in Chapter 1. TEE is therefore not needed in the majority of these conditions. TEE may be useful in the small subset of patients with aortic steno-

TABLE 6.3. Suggested Indications of TEE in Selected Patients with Prosthetic Valve Obstruction

---

Nondiagnostic or difficult transthoracic study.

Assessment of concomitant regurgitation in mild or moderate stenosis of a prosthetic mitral valve.

Selected patients with moderate stenosis (substantiate diagnosis and assess for possible reversible mechanism).

Selected patients with known severe obstruction:
  a. Candidates for thrombolysis
  b. Pre–balloon valvuloplasty for bioprosthetic valves
  c. Suspected endocarditis

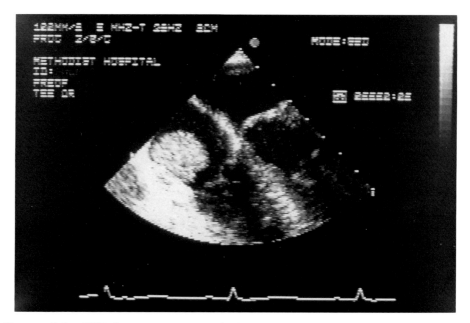

Figure 6.9. TEE showing a mass attached to the anterior wall of the right atrium. At surgery, this was proven to be an atypical myxoma.

sis who are difficult to evaluate with surface echocardiography. On the other hand, TEE is indicated in symptomatic patients with mild to moderate mitral stenosis to evaluate the severity of concomitant mitral regurgitation and in those with severe mitral stenosis, prior to balloon valvuloplasty, to exclude the presence of atrial thrombi.[46]

Cardiac Masses

Transthoracic echocardiography is an excellent modality for the diagnosis of atrial myxoma, ventricular thrombi, and tumors. With the increased resolution of TEE imaging and its better definition of the cardiac base, TEE has proven to be superior for localization and characterization of cardiac masses[47] (Figure 6.9). The technique provides structural details of the mass and its site of attachment as well as information regarding compression or infiltration of adjacent structures, features that can be helpful in differentiating malignant from benign masses. The important role of TEE in identification of left atrial and particularly left atrial appendage thrombi has been discussed earlier. The advent of biplane and multiplane TEE has facilitated visualization of the superior vena cava and improved the definition of masses in these areas, including thrombi attached to pacemaker wires or intravenous lines. With adequate visualization of the main pulmonary artery and its proximal branches, TEE can also be used for detection of large pulmonary emboli in these arteries.

Diseases of the Aorta

Segments of the aorta including the aortic root, proximal ascending aorta, portions of the arch, and proximal descending aorta can be evaluated with surface echocardiography. Although the size of the aorta at these levels can be measured, a detailed evaluation particularly as to the presence of a dissection may be limited, especially in the descending aorta. TEE has significantly improved the accuracy of ultrasound techniques in the assessment of the aorta, particularly the descending thoracic aorta. Visualization of the descending aorta is possible from the level of the stomach to the aortic arch. On the other hand, evaluation of the ascending aorta is possible from the aortic valve to the beginning of the aortic arch. Because of the interposition of the trachea between the ascending aorta and the esophagus, transesophageal imaging is limited in assessing a small portion of the distal ascending aorta/proximal arch.[3] With the recent addition of the longitudinal imaging plane, visualization of this portion of the ascending aorta has been improved.[4] Furthermore, dissection or aneurysm limited only to this portion of the aorta is in itself rare.

In patients with aortic dissection, performance of a TEE has been found to be safe. Administration of analgesics and sedatives before the procedure allows easy introduction of the probe and helps reduce the increase in blood pressure during the procedure. Using TEE, aortic dissection is identified by the presence within the aorta of two lumens separated by an intimal flap (Figure 6.10). Not infrequently, sponta-

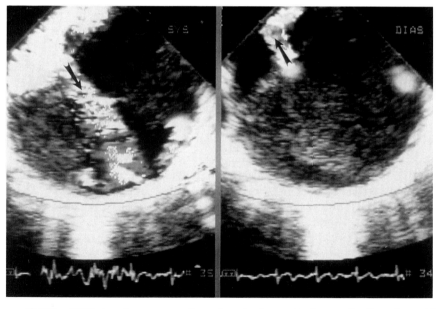

Figure 6.10.   TEE showing cross-section of aorta demonstrating aortic dissection with a true lumen and false lumen. In systole (left panel), the entry jet (arrow) is directed from the true lumen to the false lumen. The false lumen also exhibits spontaneous echo contrast, a marker of stasis. In diastole (right panel), reversal of the jet occurs from the false lumen to the true lumen as illustrated by arrow.

neous echocardiographic contrast, a marker of blood stasis, can be visualized in the false lumen with or without thrombus formation. The sensitivity and specificity of TEE for detection and classification of aortic dissection is comparable to or even better than that of more traditional imaging modalities (angiography, computed tomography [CT]).[48–51] Evaluation of concomitant aortic insufficiency, ventricular function, and the presence of pericardial effusion, important findings in patients with suspected dissection, are also readily obtainable. For any imaging modality, difficulties still exist in a small number of patients where the dissection is very small, with a hematoma formation at the site of the intimal tear. In these situations, an increase in aortic wall thickness by TEE is usually seen and may be a helpful sign. False-positive diagnoses for dissection by echocardiography are rare but can be made as a result of reverberations within the aorta.[52] Similar artifacts can also be seen with transthoracic imaging. Because of its diagnostic accuracy and portability, TEE is currently used in several centers as the first-line diagnostic imaging modality in patients with suspected aortic dissection. As previously mentioned, the importance of TEE in the evaluation of the aorta for extensive atherosclerosis and thrombi as a possible source of vascular events has been recently recognized.

Critically Ill Patients

In critically ill patients, prompt and accurate diagnostic evaluation that directs appropriate therapeutic intervention has significant impact on morbidity and mortality. However, because of the overall general condition of these patients, coupled with their inherent instability and multiple instrumentation, their transportation to different diagnostic areas can be a major endeavor. Furthermore, the choice of the diagnostic and therapeutic modality can be challenging. Echocardiography has been very popular in the intensive care units as a noninvasive and portable diagnostic modality that provides structural, functional, and hemodynamic information about the cardiovascular system. However, the adequacy and accuracy of transthoracic echocardiography in this setting may be hampered since many patients are mechanically ventilated, connected with several monitors and life-saving devices or are in the postoperative phase with recent surgical wounds. TEE overcomes several of the above limitations and has been demonstrated to be a powerful and yet safe diagnostic modality to assess the cardiovascular system in the critically ill patient.[44,45]

The insertion of a transesophageal echocardiography probe in critically ill patients requires more experience and caution. Because of the underlying clinical condition, many patients cannot cooperate with the procedure or are frequently not fully responsive. Several may be agitated and require heavy sedation. Many of these patients have an endotrachial tube and a nasogastric tube. The procedure may in some cases have to be performed with the patient in the supine position instead of the lateral decubitus position. Technical aspects of TEE in critically ill patients have been previously described.[44,45] In rare cases, the assistance of an anesthesiologist for insertion of the probe under direct visualization may be needed. During the procedure, continuous monitoring of ECG, blood pressure, and O_2 saturation is needed to enhance safety. Despite the critical status of these patients, clinically significant complications have been rare in our experience as well as with others.

TABLE 6.4. Indications of TEE in Critically Ill Patients

Suboptimal or nondiagnostic transthoracic study
Hemodynamic instability, especially without obvious cardiac cause
Valvular regurgitation, especially mitral regurgitation
Suspected endocarditis/abscess
Suspected prosthetic valve dysfunction
Postinfarct complications
Hemodynamic instability, after cardiac surgery
Aortic dissection
Cardiac contusion, potential heart donor
Source of embolism
Pericardial disease
Wearning from cardiac support devices

There are several indications for the use of TEE in the intensive care unit (Table 6.4). These include general categories such as hemodynamic instability, suspected endocarditis, suspected embolic events, and suspected aortic dissection. We have recently evaluated the diagnostic impact of TEE in 77 critically ill patients in our institution.[45] Table 6.5 lists the underlying etiologies diagnosed by TEE in the group of patients with hemodynamic instability (Figure 6.11). The impact on management has been significant in several series including ours. This includes changes in medical therapy as well as surgical interventions, frequently performed without the need of further diagnostic workup.

Congenital Heart Disease

In infants and children with congenital heart disease, transthoracic echocardiography can usually provide high-quality images and all the necessary information to

TABLE 6.5. Summary of TEE Findings in 32 Patients with Hemodynamic Instability

TEE Finding	n (%)
Native mitral regurgitation	8 (25%)
Volume depletion	7 (22%)
Left ventricular failure	5 (16%)
Right ventricular failure	3 (9%)
Prosthetic mitral regurgitation	3 (9%)
Cardiac tamponade	3 (9%
Prosthetic valve stenosis	1 (3%)
Pericardial constriction	1 (3%)
Normal prosthetic valve and cardiac function (noncardiac)	1 (3%)
Total	32 (100%)

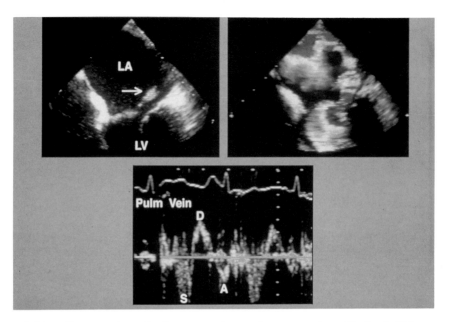

Figure 6.11. Transesophageal echo pictures in a patient presenting with shock. Echocardiographic images show a ruptured head of the papillary muscle as shown by arrow. The eccentric mitral regurgitation is depicted. Pulmonary venous flow pattern is also consistent with severe mitral regurgitation, with reversal of the systolic flows in the pulmonary veins. A = atrial reversal wave; D = diastollic wave; S = systolic reversal caused by the regurgitant jet; LA = left atrium; LV = left ventricle.

define the cardiac defects in this population. However, in certain individuals the quality of the images may be impaired. With the availability of pediatric probes, TEE currently is possible in children and even newborn infants. The procedure in the very young is usually performed under general anesthesia. TEE provides high-resolution imaging of the atrial, interatrial septum, and atrioventricular structures. It is the technique of choice to define the atrial septum and the presence of patent foramen ovale.[53,54] Sinus venosus type atrial septal defect and anomalous pulmonary venous return are detected more easily by TEE because it allows definition of each of the pulmonary veins and their drainage, which is more difficult to define with the transthoracic approach[55] (Figure 6.12). Patients with patent ductus arteriosus as well as coarctation of the aorta can be evaluated. The procedure has also been used to guide catheter-based interventions such as balloon valvuloplasty, closure of patent ductus arteriosus, or atrial septal defects with a device.

Intraoperative Use

Although surface echocardiography has been used in the operating room to assess surgical results, the advent of TEE has propelled the use of echocardiography in the operating room since it does not interfere with the surgical field. TEE has clearly been found to be beneficial in the planning of the surgical operation and evaluating the results of cardiovascular surgery.[56] The role of intraoperative TEE has been well established for valve repair where it allows immediate assessment of the operative results prior to chest closure and aids in the decision as to whether or not to under-

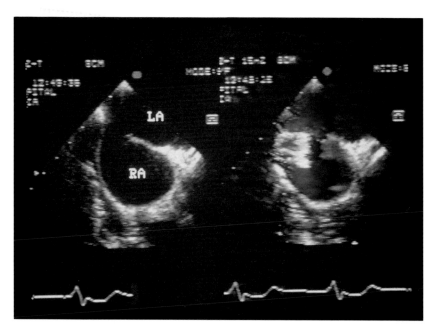

Figure 6.12.   TEE showing a sinus venosus atrial septal defect between the left atrium (LA) and the right atrium (RA). Color Doppler shows the shunt to be predominantly left to right.

take another intervention before chest closure. Moreover, TEE has also been recommended to help determine the extent of myomectomy in patients with hypertrophic cardiomyopathy and in patients undergoing repair of complex congenital heart disease.[57] TEE can also be used for cardiac monitoring. It allows the assessment of global and regional ventricular function continuously and has been shown to detect myocardial ischemia more easily with this approach than by hemodynamic evaluation.[58] It can provide assessment for hypovolemia or hypervolemia and help in weaning patients from pulmonary bypass or ventricular assist devices. Although the role of monitoring in the general surgical population is controversial, potentially this technique could be used in the high-risk individual with cardiac disease undergoing noncardiac surgery. Furthermore, TEE has been used to monitor for air or fat embolism in patients undergoing neurosurgical procedures or hip replacement.

CONTRAINDICATIONS

Prior to performance of a TEE, a careful history as to esophageal and gastric disease should be elicited. Absolute contraindications to TEE include a patient with a history of dysphasia that has not been recently investigated. A history of esophageal or gastric tumor, laceration, or recent surgery also constitute contraindications to the procedure. Relative contraindications include esophageal varices, bleeding peptic ulcer disease, severe cervical arthritis or disease. Other relative contraindications include Zenker's diverticulum, esophageal pouch, and previous surgery on the esophagus. Consultation with a gastroenterologist in these situations is prudent and a balance between the risk of the procedure and the cardiac information required needs to be evaluated.

ADVANTAGES AND DISADVANTAGES

The advantages of TEE can be surmised from the various applications mentioned above and their implication in the diagnosis and management of the cardiac patient. The fact that this methodology provides, at the bedside, excellent definition of cardiac structure, function, and associated valvular abnormalities and hemodynamics, makes TEE a unique technique in current day cardiology compared to other imaging modalities such as magnetic resonance imaging (MRI), CT scanning, or angiography. The high-resolution images obtained allow visualization of small structures such as left atrial appendage thrombi, valvular vegetations and mobile masses, and aortic debris that usually cannot be identified with other imaging modalities.

In contrast to transthoracic echocardiography, high-quality imaging is consistently obtained with TEE. Some of the disadvantages in imaging may include anterior structures in the far field, particularly if highly refractile structures are interposed, such as prosthetic valves or heavy calcifications in the mitral or aortic position. TEE in general should be regarded as a technique that complements information obtained from the transthoracic approach, particularly in these conditions. Other disadvantages of TEE include the small risk of the procedure. Experience reported from several centers including ours has shown TEE to be a safe procedure. The incidence of major complications is low and has ranged between 0.18% and 0.5%;[14,59] only two deaths have been reported. Possible other complications include hypotension, respiratory failure, hypertension, laryngospasm, atrial and ventricular arrhythmias, aspiration. The incidence of these individual minor abnormalities is, however, less than 1%.[14,59] Feasibility of the procedure is currently greater than 98% in most laboratories. To enhance the safety as well as the accuracy of TEE, it should be performed only by skilled physicians, with appropriate training in TEE.

SPECIAL CONSIDERATIONS

When used appropriately, TEE is a cost-effective modality that can have a significant impact on patient outcome and management. The cost of the procedure is in general lower than that of other diagnostic modalities in cardiology such as left or right heart catheterization, aortography, MRI, or CT scan of the thorax, when comparing the relative value units assignment by the Health Care Financing Administration.[14] With the availability of TEE, the need for cardiac catheterization to assess hemodynamics of patients with intracardiac shunts and valvular heart disease has decreased significantly. In patients with aortic dissection, TEE has replaced more conventional imaging modalities in several institutions and is frequently performed in equivocal cases of angiography or CT scans as the diagnostic modality to resolve the questionable diagnosis. Although a combination of imaging modalities may be necessary in an individual patient, the appropriate use of imaging technologies may reduce duplication of information and allow for more cost-effective care while maintaining high-quality health care delivery. In this regard, any procedure, including TEE should not be performed if the outcome or management of patients would be the same, regardless of the results of the diagnostic procedure.

FUTURE ADVANCEMENT

Within a relatively short period, TEE has seen major technological advances. Future developments are aimed at improving customized TEE probes, transducer technology, and image processing for further enhancement of image definition. Multifrequency transducer technology will allow changing frequency of the same transducer thus modifying penetration and resolution of acquired images. Innovations will also focus on improvement of transducer size while maintaining a large number of ultrasound crystals to improve resolution and increase the ease of passage of the probe and comfort to patients. Furthermore, image acquisition and processing will improve to allow three-dimensional reconstruction of echocardiographic images. Refinement of the technology will also be incorporated with other advancement in echocardiography including conversion from video to digital technology, thus eliminating degradation of images, facilitating review of serial studies, and transferring images from the laboratory to various viewing stations.

SUMMARY AND CONCLUSION

TEE currently provides a powerful diagnostic tool for clinical decision making in the cardiac patient. It has tremendously improved the diagnostic potential of transthoracic echocardiography and in certain disease entities, has eliminated the need of further diagnostic evaluation. While transthoracic echocardiography remains the primary technique for cardiac evaluation with ultrasound, TEE is indicated in several conditions to further define cardiac structure and function and diseases of the aorta and complements the transthoracic evaluation. As an invasive procedure, TEE is associated with low but identifiable risk and therefore should only be performed by skilled trained physicians in selected patients where findings may alter clinical management of patients with cardiovascular disease.

REFERENCES

1. Frazin L, Talano JV, Stephanides L, et al: Esophageal echocardiography. *Circulation* 54:102–108, 1976.
2. Souquet J, Hanrath P, Zitelli L, et al: Transesophageal phased array for imaging the heart. *IEEE Trans Biomed Eng* 29:707–712, 1982.
3. Seward JB, Khandheria BK, Oh JK, et al: Transesophageal echocardiography: tech-

nique, anatomic correlations, implementation, and clinical applications. *Mayo Clin Proc* 63:649–680, 1988.

4. Seward JB, Khandheria BK, Edwards WD, et al: Biplanar transesophageal echocardiography: anatomic correlations, image orientation, and clinical applications. *Mayo Clin Proc* 65:1193–1213, 1990.

5. Bansal RC, Shakudo M, Shah PM: Biplane transesophageal echocardiography: technique, image orientation, and preliminary experience in 131 patients. *J Am Soc Echocardiogr* 3:348–366, 1990.

6. Flachskampf FA, Hoffmann R, Verlande M, et al: Initial experience with a multiplane transesophageal echo-transducer: assessment of diagnostic potential. *Eur Heart J* 13:1201–1206, 1992.

7. Seward JB, Khandheria BK, Freeman WK, et al: Multiplane transesophageal echocardiography image orientation, examination techniques, anatomic correlations and clinical applications. *Mayo Clin Proc* 68:523–551, 1993.

8. Steckelberg JM, Khandheria BK, Anhalt JP, et al: Prospective evaluation of the risk of bacteremia associated with transesophageal echocardiography. *Circulation* 84:177–180, 1991.

9. Melendez LJ, Chan KL, Cheung PK, et al: Incidence of bacteremia in transesophageal echocardiography: prospective study of 140 consecutive patients. *J Am Coll Cardiol* 18:1650–1654, 1991.

10. Daniel WG, Mugge A: Transesophageal echocardiography. [Review]. *N Engl J Med* 332:1268–1279, 1995.

11. Khandheria BK: Prophylaxis or no prophylaxis before transesophageal echocardiography? *J Am Soc Echocardiogr* 5:285–287, 1992.

12. Pearlman AS, Gardin JM, Martin RP, et al: Guidelines for physician training in transesophageal echocardiography: recommendations of the American Society of Echocardiography Committee for Physician Training in Echocardiography. *J Am Soc Echocardiogr* 5:187–194, 1992.

13. Seward JB, Khandheria BK, Oh JK, et al: Critical appraisal of transesophageal echocardiography: limitations, pitfalls, and complications. *J Am Soc Echocardiogr* 5:288–305, 1992.

14. Khandheria BK, Seward JB, Tajik AJ: Transesophageal echocardiography. [Review]. *Mayo Clin Proc* 69:856–863, 1994.

15. Pop G, Sutherland GR, Koudstaal PJ, et al: Transesophageal echocardiography in the detection of intracardiac embolic sources in patients with transient ischemic attacks. *Stroke* 21:560–565, 1990.

16. Black IW, Hopkins AP, Lee LCL, et al: Role of transesophageal echocardiography in evaluation of cardiogenic embolism. *Br Heart J* 66:302–307, 1991.

17. Pearson AC, Labovitz AJ, Tatineni S, et al: Superiority of transesophageal echocardiography in detecting cardiac source of embolism in patients with cerebral ischemia of uncertain etiology. *J Am Coll Cardiol* 17:66–72, 1991.

18. Manning WJ, Silverman DI, Gordon SPF, et al: Cardioversion from atrial fibrillation without prolonged anticoagulation with use of transesophageal echocardiography to exclude the presence of atrial thrombi. *N Engl J Med* 328:750–755, 1993.

19. Castello R, Pearson AC, Labovitz AJ: Prevalence and clinical implications of atrial spontaneous contrast in patients undergoing transesophageal echocardiography. *Am J Cardiol* 65:1149–1153, 1990.

20. Daniel WG, Nellessen U, Schroder E, et al: Left atrial spontaneous echo contrast in mitral valve disease: an indicator for an increased thromboembolic risk. *J Am Coll Cardiol* 11:1204–1211, 1988.

21. Karalis DG, Chandrasekaran K, Victor M, et al: Recognition and embolic potential of intraaortic atherosclerotic debris. *J Am Coll Cardiol* 17:73–78, 1991.

22. Daniel WG: Should transesophageal echocardiography be used to guide cardioversion? *N Engl J Med* 328:803–804, 1993.

23. Black IW, Fatkin D, Sagar KB, et al: Exclusion of atrial thrombus by transesophageal echocardiography does not preclude embolism after cardioversion of atrial fibrillation. *Circulation* 89:2509–2513, 1994.

24. Manning WJ, Leeman DE, Gotch PJ, et al: Pulsed Doppler evaluation of atrial mechanical function after electrical cardioversion of atrial fibrillation. *J Am Coll Cardiol* 13: 617–623, 1989.

25. Manning WJ, Silverman DI, Katz SE, et al: Impaired left atrial mechanical function after cardioversion: relation to the duration of atrial fibrillation. *J Am Coll Cardiol* 23:1535–1540, 1994.

26. Mugge A, Daniel WG, Frank G, et al: Echocardiography in infective endocarditis: reassessment of prognostic implications of vegetation size determined by the transthoracic and the transesophageal approach. *J Am Coll Cardiol* 14:631–638, 1989.

27. Shively BK, Gurule FT, Roldan CA, et al: Diagnostic value of transesophageal compared with transthoracic echocardiography in infective endocarditis. *J Am Coll Cardiol* 18: 391–397, 1991.

28. Lowry RW, Zoghbi WA, Baker WB, et al: Clinical impact of transesophageal echocardiography in the diagnosis and management of infective endocarditis. *Am J Cardiol* 73: 1089–1091, 1994.

29. Daniel WG, Mugge A, Martin RP, et al: Improvement in the diagnosis of abscesses associated with endocarditis by transesophageal echocardiography. *N Engl J Med* 324:795–800, 1991.

30. Karalis DG, Bansal RC, Hauck AJ, et al: Transesophageal echocardiographic recognition of subaortic complications in aortic valve endocarditis: clinical and surgical implications. *Circulation* 86:353–362, 1992.

31. Afridi I, Apostolidou MA, Saad RM, et al: Pseudoaneurysms of the mitral-aortic intervalvular fibrosa: dynamic characterization using transesophageal echocardiographic and Doppler techniques. *J Am Coll Cardiol* 25:137–145, 1995.

32. Bansal RC, Graham BM, Jutzy KR, et al: Left ventricular outflow tract to left atrial communication secondary to rupture of mitral-aortic intervalvular fibrosa in infective endocarditis: diagnosis by transesophageal echocardiography and color flow imaging. *J Am Coll Cardiol* 15:499–504, 1990.

33. Daniel LB, Grigg LE, Weisel RD, et al: Comparison of transthoracic and transesophageal assessment of prosthetic valve dysfunction. *Echocardiography* 7:83–95, 1990.

34. Daniel WG, Mugge A, Grote J, et al: Comparison of transthoracic and transesophageal echocardiography for detection of abnormalities of prosthetic and bioprosthetic valves in the mitral and aortic positions. *Am J Cardiol* 71:210–215, 1993.

35. Zoghbi WA, Afridi I: Aortic regurgitation. In: *Current Diagnosis and Treatment in Cardiology.* East Norwalk, Appleton & Lange, 1995, pp. 99–109.

36. Barbetseas J, Crawford ES, Safi HJ, et al: Doppler echocardiographic evaluation of pseudoaneurysms complicating composite grafts of the ascending aorta. *Circulation* 85:212–222, 1992.

37. Reisner SA, Meltzer RS: Normal values of prosthetic valve Doppler echocardiographic parameters: a review. *J Am Soc Echocardiogr* 1:201–210, 1988.

38. Bitar JN, Lechin ME, Salazar G, et al: Doppler echocardiographic assessment with the continuity equation of St. Jude Medical mechanical prostheses in the mitral valve position. *Am J Cardiol* 76:287–293, 1995.

39. Chafizadeh ER, Zoghbi WA: Doppler echocardiographic assessment of the St. Jude Medical prosthetic valve in the aortic position using the continuity equation. *Circulation* 83:213–223, 1991.

40. Zoghbi WA, Desir RM, Rosen L, et al: Doppler echocardiography: application to the assessment of successful thrombolysis of prosthetic valve thrombosis. *J Am Soc Echocardiogr* 2:98–101, 1989.

41. Gueret P, Vignon P, Fournier P, et al: Transesophageal echocardiography for the diagnosis and management of nonobstructive thrombosis of mechanical mitral valve prosthesis. *Circulation* 91:103–110, 1995.

42. Dzavik V, Cohen G, Chan KL: Role of transesophageal echocardiography in the diagnosis and management of prosthetic valve thrombosis. *J Am Coll Cardiol* 18:1829–1833, 1991.

43. Himelman RB, Kusumoto F, Oken K, et al: The flail mitral valve: echocardiographic findings by precordial and transesophageal imaging and Doppler color flow mapping. *J Am Coll Cardiol* 17:272–279, 1991.

44. Oh JK, Seward JB, Khandheria BK, et al: Transesophageal echocardiography in critically ill patients. *Am J Cardiol* 66:1492–1495, 1990.

45. Khoury AF, Afridi I, Quiñones MA, et al: Transesophageal echocardiography in critically ill patients: feasibility, safety, and impact on management. *Am Heart J* 127:1363–1371, 1994.

46. Kronzon I, Tunick PA, Glassman E, et al: Transesophageal echocardiography to detect atrial clots in candidates for percutaneous transseptal mitral balloon valvuloplasty. *J Am Coll Cardiol* 16:1320–1322, 1990.

47. Mugge A, Daniel WG, Haverich A, et al: Diagnosis of noninfective cardiac mass lesions by two-dimensional echocardiography: comparison of the transthoracic and transesophageal approaches. *Circulation* 83:70–78, 1991.

48. Erbel R, Engberding R, Daniel W, et al: Echocardiography in diagnosis of aortic dissection. *Lancet* 1:456–460, 1989.

49. Ballal RS, Nanda NC, Gatewood R, et al: Usefulness of transesophageal echocardiography in assessment of aortic dissection. *Circulation* 84:1903–1914, 1991.

50. Nienaber CA, von Kodolitsch Y, Nicolas V, et al: The diagnosis of thoracic aortic dissection by noninvasive imaging procedures. *N Engl J Med* 328:1–9, 1993.

51. Light LH: Non-injurious ultrasonic technique for observing flow in the human aorta. *Nature (Lond)* 224:1119–1121, 1969.

52. Appelbe AF, Walker PG, Yeoh JK, et al: Clinical significance and origin of artifacts in transesophageal echocardiography of the thoracic aorta. *J Am Coll Cardiol* 21:754–760, 1993.

53. Mehta RH, Helmcke F, Nanda NC, et al: Transesophageal Doppler color flow mapping assessment of atrial septal defect. *J Am Coll Cardiol* 16:1010–1016, 1990.

54. Chenzbraun A, Pinto FJ, Schnittger I: Biplane transesophageal echocardiography in the diagnosis of patent foramen ovale. *J Am Soc Echocardiogr* 6:417–421, 1993.

55. Kronzon I, Tunick PA, Freedberg RS, et al: Transesophageal echocardiography is superior to transthoracic echocardiography in diagnosis of sinus venous atrial septal. *J Am Coll Cardiol* 17:537–542, 1991.

56. Sheikh KH, de Bruijn NP, Rankin JS, et al: The utility of transesophageal echocardiography and Doppler color flow imaging in patients undergoing cardiac valve surgery. *J Am Coll Cardiol* 15:363–372, 1990.

57. Grigg LE, Wigle ED, Williams WG, et al: Transesophageal Doppler echocardiography in obstructive hypertrophic cardiomyopathy: clarification of pathophysiology and importance in intraoperative decision making. *J Am Coll Cardiol* 20:42–52, 1992.
58. van Daele MERM, Sutherland GR, Mitchell MM, et al: Do changes in pulmonary capillary wedge pressure adequately reflect myocardial ischemia during anesthesia? A correlative preoperative hemodynamic, electrocardiographic, and transesophageal echocardiographic study. *Circulation* 81:865–871, 1990.
59. Daniel WG, Erbel R, Kasper W, et al: Safety of transesophageal echocardiography: a multicenter survey of 10,419 examinations. *Circulation* 83:817–821, 1991.

— Section 3 —
INVASIVE DIAGNOSTIC PROCEDURES

— 7 —

Coronary Doppler Flow Measurements

Morton J. Kern, M.D.

DESCRIPTION OF TECHNIQUE

Intracoronary Doppler flow velocity in patients can be measured with a Doppler tipped angioplasty guidewire in the cardiac catheterization laboratory. It provides an objective, physiologic measurement of coronary blood flow on which to base treatment decisions, especially important for angiographic findings of intermediate or indeterminate severity. This technique employs an angioplasty guidewire with a miniature Doppler transducer attached to its tip yielding precise spectral coronary flow velocity, measured in the distal region of the vessel, where coronary blood flow is most affected by a stenosis (Figure 7.1). Directly measured coronary blood flow velocity using the Doppler flow wire is an alternative to out of laboratory ischemic stress testing. Decisions for interventions then can be made at the time of initial angiography when stress testing has not or cannot be performed. This approach has important clinical and economic implications for patients undergoing evaluation of coronary artery disease.

DEVELOPMENTAL PERSPECTIVES

Although used as the gold standard for determination of the presence of coronary artery disease, angiography cannot determine the clinical importance of coronary stenoses narrowed between 40% and 70–80% diameter.[1] Because of this limitation, physiologic testing is often performed before deciding whether to proceed with angioplasty for patients with only angiographic findings and subjective chest pain

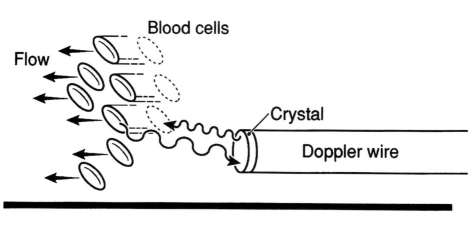

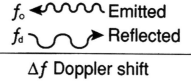

Figure 7.1. Diagram of the Doppler principle. The frequency of emitted sound is reflected off the moving red cells producing a lower reflected frequency proportional to the target velocity. This change in frequency is the Doppler shift and can be computed from the formula. Reproduced with permission from Kern et al. Ref. 13.

syndromes. Decisions regarding intracoronary interventions should be based on objective evidence of lesion severity with ischemic stress testing, such as thallium perfusion scintigraphy or abnormal lesional hemodynamics. Although coronary blood flow, coronary flow reserve, and regional perfusion have demonstrated predictable relationships between the anatomic and physiologic parameters in experimental studies, clinical reliable physiologic relationships are not present among angiography, myocardial perfusion scintigraphy, coronary flow reserve, or transstenotic pressure gradients in patients.

Doppler catheter blood flow studies have been of limited value because flow velocity data acquired proximal to the stenosis are dependent on lesion resistance with prelesional branches directing flow away from or around the lesion. Proximally measured coronary flow reserve may be nearly normal, despite severe or total occlusions when branch flow hyperemia is maintained. Prestenotic flow velocity variables, including flow reserve, have not been generally indicative of the severity of intermediate coronary stenoses.

Until recently, Doppler flow velocity has not been incorporated into routine practice because of relatively large catheters, flow measured only proximal to a stenosis, and technical difficulties in acquiring data during interventions. The Doppler guidewire has overcome catheter limitations, making it suitable for routine clinical use. Coronary flow velocity can be measured distal to a coronary stenosis and does not interfere with normal blood flow. The Doppler guidewire can be used as a primary interventional guidewire, and can monitor flow following angioplasty. Spectral

TABLE 7.1. Clinical Uses of Intravascular Doppler Coronary Flow Velocity

1. Intermediate (40–70%) lesion assessment
2. Angioplasty
   Endpoint
   Monitoring complications
   Assessing additional lesions
   Collateral flow
   Stent
   Atherectomy
3. Coronary vasodilatory reserve
   Syndrome X
   Transplant coronary arteriopathy
   Saphenous vein graft, internal mammary artery
4. Coronary research
   Pharmacologic studies
   Intra-aortic balloon pumping
   Coronary physiology of vascular disease
   Myocardial perfusion imaging correlations

Doppler signal analysis improves the operator confidence of accurate measurements. During diagnostic angiography, translesional flow can determine the hemodynamic significance of an intermediately severe (40–70%) angiographic lesion for interventional decision making.[2,3] During multivessel angioplasty, secondary lesions can be assessed before undergoing additional interventions.

The clinical applications of intracoronary flow velocity measurements are summarized in Table 7.1.

TECHNICAL CONSIDERATIONS

The Doppler Guidewires

As described and validated by Doucette et al,[4] the Doppler angioplasty guidewire (Flowire; Cardiometrics, Inc., Mountain View, CA) is a 175-cm-long, 0.018″-diameter flexible steerable guidewire with a piezoelectric ultrasound transducer integrated into the tip (Figure 7.2). The forward directed ultrasound beam diverges in a 27° arc from the long axis. The system is coupled to a real time spectrum analyzer, videocassette recorder, and video page printer. The quadrature/Doppler audio signals are processed by the spectrum analyzer and available on a scrolling gray scale video display.

Doppler Technique and Method of Use

Catheterization lab physicians can measure blood flow velocity in individual coronary arteries beyond stenoses with relative ease and safety using the Doppler velocity guidewire. The set-up time of the Flowire system is usually <10 min.

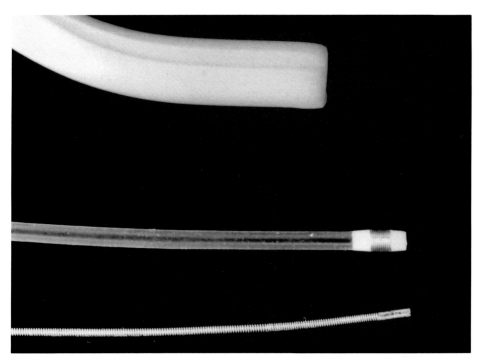

Figure 7.2. (*From top to bottom*) 8 French angiographic catheter, 2.2 French Tracker catheter (Target Therapeutics) for pressure gradient measurements, Doppler Flowire, 0.014″ (Cardiometrics, Inc., Mountain View, CA). From Ofili et al. Ref. 14.

Intravenous heparin (5,000–10,000 unit bolus) is required before inserting the Doppler guidewire. After diagnostic angiography or during angioplasty, the Doppler guidewire is passed through an angioplasty Y-connector attached to a small guiding catheter. The guidewire is then advanced into the artery. Baseline flow velocity data are obtained at least 1 cm proximal to the lesion. The guidewire is then advanced at least 5–10 artery-diameter lengths (>2 cm) beyond the stenosis and distal flow velocity data are then obtained. When velocity data are desired beyond a stenosis in the highly tortuous artery, a guidewire is advanced through a 2.7 Fr Tracker catheter, and the target lesion is crossed with the smaller guidewire; the Tracker catheter is advanced distally, the Doppler wire is then exchanged and the Tracker catheter is withdrawn.

Coronary flow velocity reserve or coronary vasodilator reserve (CVR) is computed as the quotient of hyperemic and basal mean flow velocity (Figure 7.3). Coronary hyperemia is induced by intracoronary adenosine (6–8 μg in the right coronary artery and 12–18 μg in the left coronary artery).

Although earlier studies report a CVR ratio of 3.5–5 in normal patients, in our and other laboratories, lower values are more commonly observed in patients with chest pain syndromes and angiographically normal arteries (mean coronary vasodilatory reserve ratio, 2.7 ± 0.6). In transplanted hearts with angiographic normal arteries, coronary vasodilatory reserve ratios are usually higher (3.1 ± 0.6). It should be noted that in arteries with severe coronary lesions, proximally measured flow velocity can produce nearly normal hyperemia due to augmentation of branch vessel flow. For significant stenoses, distal flow velocity reserve is always impaired (<2.0).

The Doppler guidewire can be used as the primary guidewire during routine angioplasty in >85% of attempts. Technical limitations of signal acquisition include poor guidewire tip positioning which may obscure the post-stenotic velocity. An operator examining an unsatisfactory velocity signal may falsely conclude that a velocity gradient is present.

Criteria of a Hemodynamically Significant Lesion

The use of flow velocity to assess hemodynamics of a coronary stenosis is based on the concept that the coronary circulation is comprised of two major components, a conduit (epicardial arteries) and a microcirculation (capillary and myocardial vascular

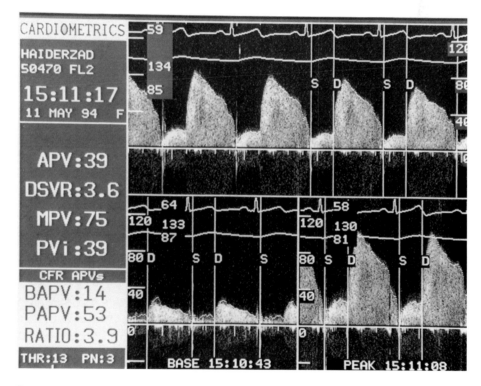

A

Figure 7.3. (A) Normal coronary flow velocity signals. The display screen is split into top and bottom which is then subdivided into left and right panels. *Top section:* Continuous phasic flow velocity during hyperemia. The velocity scale is 0–120 cm/sec. Electrocardiogram and arterial pressure are the top two tracings. S and D indicate systolic and diastolic periods. The heart rate and systolic and diastolic pressures are shown as the numbers in the gray box at the upper left corner of the flow panel. *BOTTOM left and right panels:* Coronary flow velocity at baseline and at peak hyperemia are shown in the lower panel of the split screen. The same velocity scale is used in the upper panel. APV = average peak velocity; DSVR = diastolic/systolic velocity ratio; MPV = maximal peak velocity; PVi = peak velocity integral. Coronary vasodilatory reserve is calculated from basal average peak velocity (BAPV) of 14 cm/sec and peak average peak velocity (PAPV) of 53 cm/sec to produce a coronary vasodilatory reserve ratio of 3.9 (*shown in the lower far left light gray panel*).

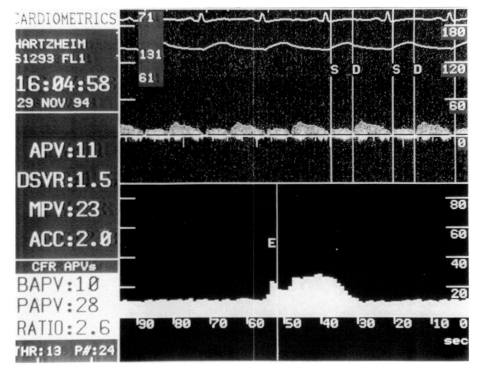

B

Figure 7.3. (B) Coronary flow velocity is also displayed as a continuous plot of the average peak velocity (*lower panel of split screen*). The trend plot scale of average peak velocity is from 0–80 cm/sec. The time divisions are 10 sec. The vertical line marked E is the event marker for injection of intracoronary adenosine. The trend plot shows coronary hyperemia after adenosine peaking at 30 sec and rapidly returning to baseline. The coronary reserve in this individual was 2.6 (abbreviations as in Figure 7.3A).

bed). If post-stenotic vasodilatory flow reserve is normal, then both components are assumed to be normal. If coronary vasodilator reserve is abnormal, then examination of lesion-specific indices will separate conduit obstruction which can be treated mechanically (angioplasty) from microcirculatory disturbances which are treated medically.

A hierarchy of findings can be used to characterize a hemodynamically and clinically significant lesion (Figure 7.4).

Post-stenotic Coronary Flow Reserve <2.0

Excellent correlations with myocardial perfusion imaging and post-stenotic coronary flow reserve have been reported by several single-center studies and one large multicenter trial. Miller et al.[5] studied 33 patients to correlate stress myocardial perfusion imaging with post-stenotic coronary flow reserve in patients with angiographically intermediate coronary stenoses. The mean angiographic percent diameter stenosis by quantitative coronary angiography was 56 ± 14% (range 20–84% diameter stenosis). Proximal and post-stenotic Doppler flow velocities were obtained at

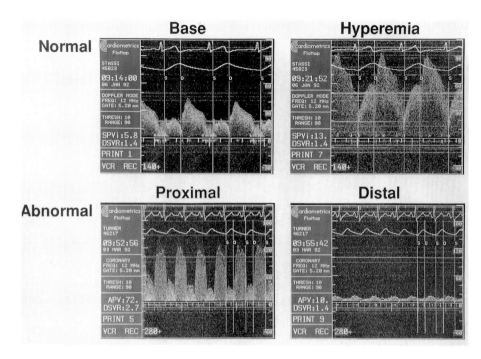

Figure 7.4. Typical flow velocity signals depicting normal hyperemia and abnormal loss of distal flow with reduction of the proximal to distal ratio, the diastolic to systolic velocity ratio, and coronary hyperemia. Format as in Figure 7.3.

rest and during maximal hyperemia induced with intracoronary adenosine.[2] Intravenous pharmacologic stress imaging was performed with adenosine in 20 patients and dipyridamole in 13 patients with technetium-99m sestamibi tomographic perfusion imaging within 1 wk of coronary flow velocity studies. A Kappa statistic measuring the strength of correlation among the velocity imaging and quantitative coronary angiographic variables was computed. Quantitative coronary angiographic stenosis severity (>50% diameter stenosis) and post-stenotic coronary flow velocity reserve of <2.0 were correlated in 20 of 27 patients (74%, $\kappa = 0.48$). Perfusion imaging abnormalities and quantitative coronary angiographic stenosis severity were correlated in 28 of 33 patients (85%, $\kappa = 0.63$). Sestamibi imaging results agreed with basal transstenotic velocity ratios (normal <1.7, abnormal >1.7) in 48% of patients ($\kappa = 0.17$). The strongest correlation was noted between hyperemic post-stenotic flow velocity reserve and sestamibi perfusion imaging in 24 of 27 patients (89%, $\kappa = 0.78$). Nearly all patients with abnormal distal hyperemic flow velocity values had corresponding reversible myocardial perfusion tomographic imaging defects. A similar correspondence between post-stenotic coronary flow reserve and myocardial perfusion imaging has been described by Joye et al.[6]

The high correlation between two different physiologic techniques to assess myocardial perfusion in the post-stenotic region suggests that clinical decisions can be made in the laboratory in a fashion similar to out-of-laboratory testing. The physiologic assessment of coronary stenoses, especially those of angiographically intermediate severity, may be improved by the use of post-stenotic flow velocity measurements when perfusion imaging has not or cannot be performed.

These studies indicate that post-stenotic flow reserve can perform in a manner similar to myocardial perfusion imaging in the assessment of coronary stenoses. In accepting the limitations of both techniques, decisions for intervention based on myocardial perfusion imaging can be extended to post-stenotic coronary vasodilatory reserve.

Lesion-specific Indices

Proximal To Distal Flow Velocity Ratio <1.7. Distal coronary flow velocity is lower than proximal flow velocity in a branched artery in proportion to the resistance imparted by the stenosis to translesional flow. This ratio is related to the pressure loss across a stenosis. Donohue et al.[2] first described this index in a study of 88 patients during diagnostic coronary angiography measuring translesional flow and pressure as described above.

There was a strong correlation between translesional pressure gradients and the ratios of the proximal to distal total flow velocity integrals ($r = 0.8$, $p < 0.001$) with a weaker relationship between quantitative angiography and pressure gradients ($r = 0.6$, $p < 0.001$). In angiographically intermediate stenoses (range 50–70%), angiography was a poor predictor of translesional gradients ($r = 0.2$, $p = $ NS) while the flow velocity ratios continued to have a strong correlation ($r = 0.8$, $p < 0.0001$). This flow ratio demonstrated highly significant differences between pressure gradients <20 mm Hg (group 1) or >20 mm Hg (group 2), ranging from 1.1 ± 0.3 for group 1 to ranges of 2.4 ± 0.9 to 2.5 ± 1.2 for group 2 $p < 0.001$ versus group 1). In 17 normal patients and 29 patients with angiographic percent stenoses ranging from 50% to 85% and translesional gradients from 0 to 85 mm Hg, CVR in the normal arteries was 2.5 ± 0.7 proximally and 2.6 ± 0.6 in the distal portion of the artery. In the diseased vessels, the proximally measured coronary flow reserve was not significantly different for any translesional gradient and could not distinguish between stenoses with gradients <20 mm Hg (2.1 ± 0.7) versus those > 20 mm Hg (1.7 ± 0.6, $p = $ NS). The coronary flow reserve measured distal to the area of stenosis was able to differentiate between these two groups with a distal coronary flow reserve of 2.1 ± 0.7 in those with gradients <20 mm Hg and 1.4 ± 0.6 ($p < 0.01$) in those with gradients > 20 mm Hg.

A proximal to distal flow velocity integral ratio of <1.7 was associated with a gradient <30 mm Hg in >85% of patients. Patients with nonbranching right coronary artery lesions had normal proximal to distal flow velocity ratios despite high translesional gradients. Decremental distal flow relative to proximal flow is predicated on a branched tube model, wherein flow is diverted away from the branch with a high resistance (stenosis) to branches with lower resistances. The proximal/distal ratio will not apply in single tubes without branches where the continuity equation mandates equality of flow at any point along the circuit. In arteries that are single-tube conduits without branches, such as very proximal right coronary artery or in bypass grafts, the proximal and distal blood flow velocity will be affected equally as determined by the continuity equation. This index is sensitive but not specific for a translesional gradient.

The Diastolic To Systolic Velocity Ratio (DSVR) is <1.8, 1.5, and 1.2 for the left anterior descending/circumflex, posterior descending, and proximal right coronary artery, respectively.[7] The phasic pattern of flow reflects stenois resistance and as a stenosis becomes more severe impairs diastolic flow first, then systolic flow.

Thus, a reduction of the normal diastolic predominance of the phasic pattern will reduce the diastolic to systolic velocity ratio. This relationship requires a normally contracting myocardium in the region of the target stenosis.

In some patients where the measurements are conflicting or have borderline values (e.g., abnormal coronary flow reserve, normal proximal to distal ratio, and DSVR), a translesional pressure gradient will eliminate ambiguity. Pressure gradients should be assessed during maximal hyperemia to compute a fractional flow reserve as noted by Pijls et al.[8]

INDICATIONS

There are three major indications for coronary Doppler flow measurements: (1) assessment of the angiographically intermediate lesion, (2) decision for angioplasty of secondary lesions in multivessel angioplasty, and (3) endpoint determination after angioplasty.[9]

Assessment of The Intermediately Severe Stenosis

There are approximately 1,000,000 coronary angiograms performed in the United States each year. In patients having coronary angiography, an intermediate stenosis (40–70% diameter narrowing) is encountered in nearly 50% of all patients. Of these patients only 50% are estimated to have stress testing to assess the need for further medical therapy or intervention. Intracoronary flow velocity measurements obtained at the time of diagnostic angiography, employing the criteria of lesion significance above, can identify important lesions and save patient cost, hospital days, and catheterization lab resources.

Deferring angioplasty of intermediate (40–70%) lesions with normal translesional hemodynamics is safe and has an excellent clinical outcome. A prospective study[3] determined the feasibility, safety, and outcome of deferring angioplasty in patients with such lesions. Translesional pressure and flow velocity data were obtained in 88 patients with 100 lesions (26 single-vessel, 74 multivessel coronary artery stenoses) scheduled for angioplasty. Patients were considered eligible for the study if there was at least one coronary narrowing >50% diameter narrowed by visual estimation in the laboratory at the time of diagnostic study. Translesional hemodynamics were measured and angioplasty was deferred if the values were normal.

The deferred angioplasty group was comprised of 88 patients, 26 patients with single vessel and 62 with multivessel coronary artery disease. Nine of 26 patients with single-vessel disease were evaluated for restenosis. Fourteen of 62 multivessel patients had angioplasty of a severe lesion with pressure–flow velocity assessed in the target lesion in another vessel.

Translesional flow velocity and pressure were measured 10 min after coronary angiography with a Doppler angioplasty guidewire and a 2.7 Fr tracking catheter. Flow data were not acquired in patients whose angiograms demonstrated left main narrowings >40%, or who had highly tortuous, small (<2.0 mm diameter), or diffusely diseased arteries.

The percent lumen area reduction, percent diameter stenosis, and obstruction diameter in the deferred group were $77 \pm 8\%$, $54 \pm 7\%$, and 1.32 ± 0.33 mm, respectively. Translesional pressure gradients were lower for the deferred compared to a reference angioplasty group (10 ± 9 versus 46 ± 22 mm Hg, $p < 0.01$). Proximal/distal velocity ratios demonstrated similar values for both the normal and deferred groups with significant differences compared to the angioplasty group (1.1 ± 0.35 for the normal, 1.3 ± 0.55 for the deferred, and 2.3 ± 1.2 for the angioplasty group; $p < 0.05$ versus both normal and deferred groups).

Clinical follow-up data was available in 84 of 88 (95%) with a mean of 10 ± 8 months; minimum follow-up period was 6 months with a range of 6 to 30 months. In the deferred group, rehospitalization due to both noncardiac and anginal-like symptoms occurred in 18 patients, 12 of whom had cardiac events. No patient had a myocardial infarction. One patient died due to postangioplasty complications of a nontarget artery. One patient with multivessel coronary artery disease and decreased left ventricular function had sudden death 12 months after lesion assessment due to ventricular fibrillation. Seven patients had repeat coronary angiography without apparent angiographic change in the target lesions where intervention was unnecessary based on negative stress testing. Ten patients required either coronary artery bypass grafting (n = 6) or coronary angioplasty (n = 4), only six of which involved target arteries. Of the six patients who required bypass surgery, only three involved a target artery with previously normal translesional flow velocity.

There were no complications related to translesional pressure or flow velocity measurements in any patient studied.

This study demonstrated that in patients with angiographically intermediately severe lesions, normal translesional hemodynamic data can be acquired safely and that angioplasty can be deferred with approximately 92% of target arteries evaluated remaining stable without the need for intervention. No patient developed acute myocardial infarction, unstable angina, or death related to progression of a target artery lesion. By visual angiographic and clinical criteria, a majority of these lesions would have been dilated, many without any physiologic assessment of lesion significance, such as ischemic stress testing. A recent retrospective review of the practice of angioplasty in the United States indicates that in >60% of patients, no objective evidence of myocardial ischemia was obtained prior to coronary interventions.[10]

The use of translesional hemodynamic data to assist the clinical decision for intervention represents a departure from current interventional cardiology practice. In-laboratory physiologic assessment may be especially important when ischemic stress testing has not or cannot be performed, or has yielded equivocal results. This approach may also assist in selecting hemodynamically significant lesions in the routine practice of multivessel/multilesion angioplasty in which not only is the assumed culprit lesion addressed, but also other angiographically significant lesions are often dilated without additional assessment.

Resting translesional hemodynamics may not reflect dynamic, ischemia-producing conditions, such as exercise or emotional stimuli, potentially associated with coronary vasoconstriction and/or increased myocardial blood flow demands, conditions readily responsive to medical therapy. Angioplasty enlargement of the epicardial arterial lumen may not improve distal flow, especially for lesions with normal resting and hyperemic flow and pressure gradients. Medical therapy to limit episodic reduction of coronary flow may account for the clinical improvement or stabilization of symptoms in the deferred angioplasty group in this and similar studies.

Translesional flow velocity–pressure measurements can provide objective functional evidence of lesion significance to assist in selecting patients for appropriate coronary interventions. It is safe to postpone angioplasty for patients who have intermediate lesions that have normal translesional hemodynamics.

Use During Angioplasty

Angioplasty is performed in a routine manner using the Flowire. During coronary balloon occlusion, flow velocity rapidly falls to near zero. If persistent antegrade flow occurs, the balloon is undersized or there is collateral input distal to the balloon but proximal to the wire tip. If flow velocity initially falls to zero then becomes visible below the baseline (negative), retrograde collateral flow is identified and can be quantitated. The presence of retrograde collateral flow velocity during occlusion occurs in 10–15% of cases and may be a useful indicator of the patient's potential tolerance for prolonged balloon occlusions.

Coronary balloon deflations are associated with an immediate postischemic hyperemic velocity, usually >2 times basal flow which equilibrates over 3–4 min to the new post–percutaneous transluminal coronary angioplasty (post-PTCA) basal level. Failure to observe post-PTCA hyperemia likely indicates continued obstruction to flow at or below the level of the angioplasty site. After angioplasty, a satisfactory result is demonstrated by normalization of CVR, increase in the distal average flow, and return of diastolic predominant phasic flow velocity (DSVR) (Figure 7.5).

Multivessel Angioplasty

Secondary lesions in multivessel coronary artery disease can be addressed at the time of angioplasty of the culprit vessel using flow velocity lesion assessment as described for the intermediate lesion. This approach has the potential to save the costs of addition hospital days, stress testing, angioplasty equipment, and complications.

Endpoint of Treatment

The preliminary results of a European multicenter prospective study DEBATE (Doppler endpoint balloon angioplasty trial Europe[12] to identify the predictive value of coronary flow velocity measurements after PTCA indicate that patients with high CVR after PTCA had fewer early and late adverse effects than patients with low CVR. There was no relationship of immediate post-PTCA CVR to angiographic restenosis using a dichotomous value definition of restenosis of >50% lumen diameter narrowing.

In the preliminary study of 108 patients undergoing single-vessel PTCA (left anterior descending or circumflex artery, n = 82 or right coronary artery, n = 26), coronary flow velocity was measured with a Doppler angioplasty guidewire at rest and after maximal hyperemia with intracoronary adenosine. Post-stenotic coronary vasodilatory reserve, proximal to distal flow ratio and diastolic to systolic flow ratio (DSVR) was compared to quantitative angiographic parameters before and after PTCA. All data were analyzed by a core laboratory and correlated to clinical outcomes of ischemia (positive exercise stress test or recurrent angina).

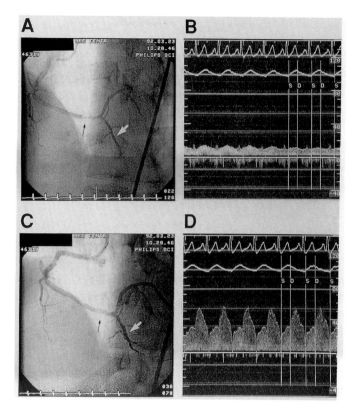

Figure 7.5. (A) Before angioplasty the right coronary artery (left anterior oblique projection) shows severe narrowing (*small black arrow*). Distal velocity is measured in the posterior descending branch (*white arrow*). (B) Abnormal distal flow velocity is evident with blunted diastolic/systolic velocity ratio and low mean velocity (10 cm/sec). Hyperemia is impaired (not shown) (C) After PTCA the angiogram shows improvement in the RCA lesion (*black arrow*). (D) Normal distal right coronary artery velocity, measured at white arrow, is characterized by normal diastolic/systolic velocity ratio and mean velocity (30 cm/sec). Reproduced with permission from Kern and Flynn. Ref. 15.

At the 30-day control, 58 of 75 (77%) patients were free of ischemic events and 17 patients (23%) either had typical chest pain (n = 10) and/or a positive electrocardiographic exercise test. The results indicated no difference in the angiographic minimal lumen diameter between the group with ischemic events and the asymptomatic patients (1.81 ± 0.39 versus 1.79 ± 0.29, p = ns). However, the post-stenotic coronary vasodilatory reserve (2.73 ± 0.93 versus 2.22 ± 0.64, p < 0.05) and the DSVR in the left anterior descending artery (LAD) (2.77 ± 1.57 versus 2.14 ± 0.69, p < 0.05) was higher in the asymptomatic compared to the ischemic event patients.

Flow velocity measurements distal to the stenosis immediately after PTCA, but not quantitative coronary angiography (QCA) data, are predictive of early ischemic events and suggest that intracoronary Doppler can identify significant residual lumen impairment which is not evident by angiography alone and which may be responsible for the increased early event rate in this group.

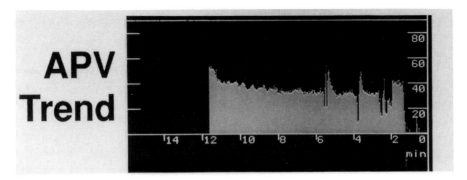

Figure 7.6. Trend of average peak velocity (APV) over a 12-min period following coronary angioplasty. This trend illustrates a stable flow pattern with a gradual decline to a stable plateau. The spikes preceded by signal loss are contrast media injections for angiography.

Monitoring Coronary Blood Flow During PTCA

Monitoring flow for variations due to slowly progressive dissection, thrombus, or vasospasm is easily performed using the mean velocity trend plot (Figure 7.6). The flow velocity trend changes often precede angiographic signs of vessel occlusion.[11] Monitoring flow can also reduce total contrast volume when assessing stability of angioplasty results and can identify potential unstable flow associated with vessel closure, a benefit which has obvious clinical advantages. Interruption of unstable flow with conversion to a stable postprocedure flow pattern reduces morbidity related to an out-of-laboratory acute vessel closure and reduces the need for a repeat procedure, angioplasty catheters, and/or stent placement. Early warning signs of an adverse outcome derived from flow trend monitoring can potentially save the cost of the repeat angioplasty and/or bypass surgery.

CONTRAINDICATIONS

The Doppler guidewire performs as an angioplasty guidewire and has an excellent safety record. In over 1,200 studies performed in our laboratory with normal or mildly diseased vessels, no patient has had a Doppler guidewire complication. Worldwide, only 10 cases out of more than 40,000 uses has resulted in serious artery injury reported to the manufacturer or FDA. This incidence is lower than diagnostic angiography alone.

Caution should be employed by operators without guidewire experience. There is no absolute contraindication to the use of intracoronary adenosine for coronary vasodilatory reserve measurements when used in the appropriate dosages. Some cardiac transplant patients may be sensitive to standard doses of adenosine which may cause transient heart block lasting <2–3 sec. Unlike papaverine, no complication has been reported with adenosine given for CVR measurements.

ADVANTAGES AND DISADVANTAGES

Intracoronary Doppler has several advantages in the assessment of coronary blood flow. It measures red blood cell velocity directly so that indicator–dilution markers are not required. Subselective Doppler guidewire insertion in distal epicardial vessels permits regional myocardial flow velocity measurements. The technique is easily incorporated into all interventional procedures using angioplasty guidewires. It can be used during diagnostic angiography without significant risk. The clinical correlations and outcome data related to coronary flow velocity indicate both economic and clinical benefit are associated with the measurements.

Technical factors involved in accurate acquisition of flow velocity signals include a stable sample volume which is undisturbed by turbulence at the lesion site. Maximal flow velocity is more accurately identified with spectral analysis due to the automatic edge detection, wide beam angle, and relative position insensitivity of the signal. The use of a guidewire rather than a catheter allows safe interrogation of smaller, more diffusely diseased arteries. Flow velocity measurements can also be performed continuously during interventional procedures providing data unavailable by catheter-based techniques.

Limitations of the Doppler guidewire are related to (1) performance as a guidewire, and (2) Doppler signal acquisition in small vessels.

The construction of the Doppler guidewire is identical to that of a normal PTCA guidewire. A 90% primary lesion crossing rate can be achieved in most laboratories. The quality of the signal and value of the peak velocity are dependent on positioning of the tip and thus may be affected by a highly distorted angle. The Doppler guidewire is durable but it may be damaged by rough handling on insertion. Manipulation within the coronary system may bend the guidewire tip but rarely is severe enough to cause signal failure. Intracoronary Doppler velocity measurements are, in part, operator-dependent. The conditions altering signal quality and accuracy should be recognized by the operator.

Problems in coronary flow velocity signal acquisition occur in <10% of patients within normal arteries and <15% of arteries examined in the course of coronary angioplasty. Occasionally it may be difficult to find the maximal distal flow velocity signals. Therefore, as performed with transthoracic echo studies, the Doppler velocity signal should be examined during several different tip orientations to interrogate maximal velocity spectra. In a region with diffuse distal disease, flow velocity acceleration may occur secondary to distal luminal narrowing. An elevated distal flow velocity may falsely normalize the proximal to distal flow velocity ratio. In patients with serial lesions or diffuse distal disease, the proximal to distal flow ratio should not be used. In these cases, confirmation of a lesion significance with coronary vasodilatory reserve and translesional pressure gradients may be needed.

SPECIAL CONSIDERATIONS

Cost savings can occur using coronary flow velocity assessment in the catheterization lab:

Preliminary data of a randomized trial conducted from physicians in Atlanta, Georgia using in-laboratory lesion assessment versus postangiography out-of-laboratory noninvasive thallium testing demonstrate substantial reduction in hospital days and total expenditure based on thallium cost estimates of $1,200.00 versus Doppler guidewire of $500.00.

FUTURE ADVANCEMENT

The decision for stent placement is expensive and commonly made from angiographic data alone. From ultrasound imaging and Doppler flow data, traditional balloon angioplasty may not achieve an optimal result for lumenal enlargement despite a satisfactory angiographic appearance. The use of stents allows a determination of the mechanism of improved coronary flow reserve after angioplasty. If residual material within the conduit lumen is responsible for abnormal CVR after PTCA, then placement of a coronary stent should normalize the CVR. These data may lead to the use of coronary flow to assist in making decisions for stenting or larger balloon catheters.

A preliminary study from our laboratory examined results in 15 patients undergoing elective angioplasty and stent placement with measurements of coronary flow velocity reserve (0.014 in Doppler flowire) and intravascular ultrasound (IVUS) imaging (2.9 F CVIS) before and after balloon angioplasty and again after stent placement.

The percent diameter stenosis decreased from $71 \pm 10\%$ to $37 \pm 11\%$ after angioplasty to $7 \pm 12\%$ after stent placement. CVR increased from 1.3 ± 0.6 to 1.6 ± 0.6 after angioplasty to 2.3 ± 0.5 after stent placement. This value was similar to that found in normal adjacent reference vessels (2.5 ± 0.6). There was no relationship between CVR and angiographic percent diameter stenosis or absolute QCA dimensions. IVUS vessel cross-sectional area was significantly larger after stenting (4.5 mm^2 after PTCA versus 7.6 mm^2 after stent, $p < 0.01$).

The increase in CVR after stenting, but not PTCA, indicates that a major mechanism of impaired CVR after angioplasty is due to inadequate lumen expansion that is not identified by angiography. These data support physiologically guided intervention to achieve an optimal lumen for flow and may lead to improved angioplasty technique to limit unnecessary stent placement.

SUMMARY

Numerous studies have shown that neither thallium testing nor angiography is sufficiently reliable to distinguish the physiologic significance of "marginal" coronary lesions. Incorporation of translesional flow velocity into clinical practice will assist in identification of appropriate angioplasty candidates and outcome of interventional procedures.

For angioplasty and similar coronary interventions, intracoronary flow velocity measurements can be used to determine the success and stability of a given result. Decisions for performing additional angioplasty are based on data identical to that used for assessing intermediate lesions. Improved clinical results after interventions appear related to final coronary flow reserve, supporting the incorporation of interventional physiology into routine practice.

REFERENCES

1. White CW, Wright CB, Doty DB, et al: Does visual interpretation of the coronary arteriogram predict the physiologic importance of a coronary stenosis? *N Engl J Med* 310:819–824, 1984.
2. Donohue TJ, Kern MJ, Aguirre FV, et al: Assessing the hemodynamic significance of coronary artery stenoses: analysis of translesional pressure–flow velocity relationships in patients. *J Am Coll Cardiol* 1993;22:449–458.
3. Kern MJ, Donohue TJ, Aguirre FV, et al: Clinical outcome of deferring angioplasty in patients with normal translesional pressure–flow velocity measurements. *J Am Coll Cardiol* 1995;25:178–187.
4. Doucette JW, Corl PD, Payne HM, et al: Validation of a Doppler guide wire for intravascular measurement of coronary artery flow velocity. *Circulation* 1992;85:1899–1911.
5. Miller DD, Donohue TJ, Younis LT, et al: Correlation of pharmacologic 99mTc-sestamibi myocardial perfusion imaging with poststenotic coronary flow reserve in patients with angiographically intermediate coronary artery stenoses. *Circulation* 1994;89: 2150–2160.
6. Joye JD, Schulman DS, Lsaorda D, et al: Intracoronary Doppler guide wire versus stress single-photon emission computed tomographic thallium-201 imaging in assessment of intermediate coronary stenoses. *J Am Coll Cardiol* 24:940–947, 1994.
7. Segal J, Kern MJ, Scott NA, et al: Alterations of phasic coronary artery flow velocity in man during percutaneous coronary angioplasty. *J Am Coll Cardiol* 1992;20:276–286.
8. Pijls NHJ, van Son AM, Kirkeeide RL, et al: Experimental basis of determining maximum coronary, myocardial, and collateral blood flow by pressure measurements for assessing functional stenosis severity before and after percutaneous transluminal coronary angioplasty. *Circulation* 1993;87:1354–1367.
9. Kern MJ, Anderson HV (eds): A symposium: the clinical applications of the intracoronary Doppler guidewire flow velocity in patients: understanding blood flow beyond the coronary stenosis. *Am J Cardiol* 71:1D–86D, 1993.
10. Topol EJ, Ellis SG, Cosgrove DM, et al: Analysis of coronary angioplasty practice in the United States with an insurance-claims data base. *Circulation* 1993;87:1489–1497.
11. Kern MJ, Donohue T, Bach R, et al: Monitoring cyclical coronary blood flow alterations following coronary angioplasty for stent restenosis using a Doppler guidewire. *Am Heart J* 1993;125:1159–1160.
12. Di Mario C, Piek JJ, Vrints C, et al for the D.E.B.A.T.E. study group. *Eur Heart J* 1995; 16:216A.
13. Kern MJ, Aguirre FV, Bach RG, et al: Interventional physiology rounds: fundamentals of translesional pressure–flow velocity measurements. *Cathet Cardiovasc Diagn* 31:137–143, 1994.
14. Ofili EO, Kern MJ, Labovitz AJ, et al: Analysis of coronary blood flow velocity dynamics in angiographically normal and stenosed arteries before and after endoluminal enlargement by angioplasty. *J Am Coll Cardiol* 1993;21:308–316.
15. Kern MJ, Flynn MS: Clinical applications of intracoronary coronary Doppler flow velocity in interventional cardiology. In White CJ, Ramee SR (eds): *Interventional Cardiology: New Technologies and Strategies for Diagnosis and Treatment.* New York, Marcel Dekker, 1995, pp 39–78.

—8—

Electrophysiologic Studies

G. Joseph Gallinghouse, M.D.
Melvin M. Scheinman, M.D.

Over the past 20 years, invasive electrophysiologic testing has evolved from diagnostic evaluation to become an indispensable tool in the treatment of cardiac arrhythmias. Initially, invasive studies were used to define the mechanisms of conduction block and arrhythmias that formerly could only be inferred from the surface electrocardiogram. Later, programmed stimulation became widely used to judge the effectiveness of antiarrhythmic drug therapy. Now this technique has become a primary therapeutic modality for several arrhythmias, and holds promise to be successfully applied to such difficult-to-treat conditions as atrial fibrillation and ischemic ventricular tachycardia.

This chapter will focus on the indications for electrophysiologic testing, with emphasis on how these studies can be expected to impact therapy.

TECHNICAL PERSPECTIVES

Invasive electrophysiologic studies are performed by positioning multipolar electrode catheters in the heart using venous and arterial approaches. Under fluoroscopic guidance, the catheters are placed at various intracardiac sites to record local electrical activity from the atria, coronary sinus, ventricles, bundle of His, and accessory pathways, if present. The myocardium is stimulated using programmed pacing. The information gathered allows for the diagnosis of conduction disturbances and arrhythmias, and provides insight into their electrophysiologic mechanisms. In recent years catheters have been developed which deliver radiofrequency energy to the tip, allowing for the safe and precise placement of burns at the endocardial surface. This technique of "radiofrequency ablation" has extended the role of invasive electrophysiology from diagnosis and prognosis to that of a primary therapeutic modality.

DEVELOPMENTAL PERSPECTIVES

Invasive electrophysiologic testing has been in clinical use since the late 1960s. Scherlag et al. published the first reports describing electrode catheter techniques to record His-bundle electrograms in 1968.[1] In the same year Durrer et al. and Coumel et al. independently reported the use of programmed electrical stimulation to induce and terminate arrhythmias.[2,3] A major advance came in 1971 with the combined use of programmed electrical stimulation with intracardiac recordings by Wellens.[4] This resulted in the rapid development of our understanding of the physiology of the conduction system, description of refractory periods in the heart, and the assessment of antiarrhythmic drugs. Multiple catheters began to be placed in the heart facilitating detailed electrical mapping, leading to localization of bypass tracts and the definition of mechanisms of supraventricular and ventricular arrhythmias.

In 1982 Scheinman et al. described the first closed chest ablation of the atrioventricular (AV) node for rate control of refractory supraventricular arrhythmias, moving invasive electrophysiology into the therapeutic era.[5] The initial energy source was direct current (DC), usually delivered from a standard cardioverter/defibrillator. This was found to be associated with arcing and barotrauma to the tissues, however, and thus produced inhomogeneous necrosis. Today radiofrequency energy (RF) using alternating current has replaced DC ablation, resulting in thermal tissue injury with focal lesions of coagulation necrosis. Advances in catheter design provide fine control of the ablation tip, allowing precise placement of burns on the endocardial surface and widening applications to multiple arrhythmias.

INDICATIONS FOR INVASIVE ELECTROPHYSIOLOGIC STUDIES

The indications for electrophysiologic studies in the evaluation of symptoms and for specific arrhythmias have undergone significant change over the past several years. The observation that traditional pharmacotherapy for ventricular arrhythmias, even when guided by invasive studies, may not offer a survival benefit over empiric therapy with amiodarone or defibrillators has had a significant impact on the role of electrophysiologic testing in these patients. On the other hand, the advent of safe and effective interventional therapy with radiofrequency ablation for many supraventricular and ventricular arrhythmias has resulted in new therapeutic indications. The fundamental goal of alleviating suffering and reducing mortality must be weighed against the costs and risks of the procedure. In this vein, a joint task force of the American College of Cardiology and the American Heart Association has recently published new guidelines for invasive testing.[6] We will describe, where appropriate, how evolving therapeutic approaches affect the indications for these procedures, and offer our perspectives on this rapidly evolving era of diagnosis and therapy for cardiac arrhythmias.

BRADYARRHYTHMIAS AND CONDUCTION ABNORMALITIES

The primary goals in the evaluation of patients with bradyarrhythmias and conduction abnormalities are to determine the location of block, to establish the relationship to symptoms, and to evaluate the likelihood of progression to high-grade heart block. It is well recognized that the prognosis of patients with bradyarrhythmias is dependent on the location of the conduction abnormality. Disease localized to the AV node generally carries a benign prognosis, whereas infranodal block portends higher risk of progression to symptomatic high-grade block. The utility of invasive testing lies in the ability both to locate the site of disease and to quantitate the magnitude of the conduction disturbance. Careful analysis of the ECG and rhythm strips allows for accurate location of the site of block and need for pacing. Invasive studies are reserved for the more difficult cases.

The diagnosis of sick sinus syndrome (sinus bradycardia, sinus arrest with junctional or ventricular escape, tachycardia–bradycardia syndrome) can generally be made noninvasively. The standard 12–lead ECG and Holter monitor are usually sufficient, relegating invasive study to a secondary role. Invasive sinus node testing is usually reserved for patients with suspected disease but where noninvasive testing is not definitive. This allows for assessment of sinus node automaticity and sinoatrial conduction.

Sinus node dysfunction is evaluated using sinus node recovery time (SNRT), which is the time from abrupt discontinuation of atrial overdrive pacing to resumption of sinus rhythm. Excessive delays in recovery of automaticity after abrupt termination of pacing usually indicate abnormal automaticity of the node. Sinoatrial conduction may also be estimated by introducing atrial extrastimuli or with atrial pacing. The low specificity of these tests has limited their usefulness in the diagnosis or treatment of this disorder.

Asymptomatic patients with sick sinus syndrome require no treatment, and thus there is no role for invasive studies. In symptomatic patients, invasive testing may provide information on the presence of associated conduction defects that might influence the type of pacemaker implanted. It should be remembered that up to 50% of patients with symptomatic sinus node disease have associated AV conduction abnormalities.[7] Also, these patients may be subject to other symptomatic arrhythmias that can be revealed invasively.

First-degree block is often the result of drug effects, and is therefore frequently reversible. It is most commonly localized to the AV node, but may be infranodal. The rate of progression to complete AV block is extremely low in asymptomatic patients with narrow or broad QRS complexes, and thus invasive evaluation is not warranted. However, patients with first-degree block who have symptoms suggestive of intermittent higher grade block (syncope, dizziness, fatigue), or concomitant arrhythmias, should undergo study if noninvasive evaluation is unable to provide a diagnosis.

The prognosis of patients with second-degree AV block is dependent on the site of block, and whether there is underlying structural heart disease. The site of block can usually be inferred from the 12-lead ECG in conjunction with vagal maneuvers or atropine, and invasive testing is not necessary for diagnosis. Type I block (Wenckebach), when associated with a narrow complex QRS, is usually located in the AV node. Type II block, on the other hand, is almost always located in or below the bundle of His. AV block that improves with vagal stimulation and associated sinus slowing implies infranodal disease. As described above, isolated AV nodal block is generally benign and usually requires no treatment, whereas infranodal disease carries higher risk. Most ominous is infra-Hisian block which is usually associated with organic heart disease, and frequently progresses to higher degrees of block with syncope or death.[8]

The decision to treat with permanent cardiac pacing is straightforward in symptomatic patients with clear evidence of second-degree AV block. Symptomatic patients with suspected His-Purkinje block should undergo invasive study. Likewise, if the site of AV block is unclear from the surface ECG, asymptomatic patients with second-degree block should be studied to identify those at high risk (intra- or infra-Hisian) for progression to complete AV block. An uncommon but interesting phenomenon that mimics second-degree AV block results from concealed retrograde conduction of junctional premature beats. This so-called "pseudo AV block" should be suspected when premature junctional beats are present, but definitive diagnosis can only be made with His bundle recordings.

As with other forms of AV conduction disorders, the lesions that produce complete AV block may occur at any level of the conduction system. Patients with block at the AV node frequently present with fatigue or dyspnea owing to bradycardia. In contrast, those with infranodal block usually present with syncope or sudden death. In these patients pacing is indicated on clinical grounds and invasive study is not necessary.

Prospective studies of patients with chronic bundle branch block show progression to complete AV block of only 1–2% per year.[9] The sudden cardiac death rate is 3–5% per year, possibly reflecting a much higher risk in this population of ventricular tachyarrhythmias than heart block. The nature of underlying cardiac pathology is obviously the critical determinant of long-term mortality in these patients.

While prophylactic pacing would be expected to benefit some patients with intraventricular conduction delay (IVCD), surface ECG findings have not been useful in defining those at risk. Presence of bi- or trifascicular block does not clearly differentiate patients with adequate sensitivity and specificity to guide therapy. Invasive HIS recordings, by accurately measuring the degree of conduction delay, seem to differentiate high-risk patients with greater accuracy.

Several studies have assessed the role of invasive studies in an attempt to improve risk stratification in this population.[9,10] Our group found that in patients with chronic bundle-branch block and abnormal H-V intervals, longer intervals conferred higher risk.[11] Patients with H-V intervals greater than or equal to 70 msec (normal 35–55 msec) had a 12% incidence of progression to second- or third-degree heart block over a 3-yr period. Those with H-V greater than or equal to 100 msec developed AV block with a 24% progression rate. Only 5% of such patients had an H-V > 100 msec, while 37% had an H-V < 70 msec.

Another study employed atrial pacing to "stress" the conduction system in an attempt to reveal occult abnormalities.[12] When AV nodal conduction was intact, those developing infranodal block with pacing progressed to second- or third-degree AV block at a rate of 14% per yr. Only 3% of patients studied had such a finding, but pacing predicted 60% of all episodes of high-grade block and/or sudden death.

Supraventricular Tachyarrhythmias

The approach to therapy of patients with supraventricular tachyarrhythmias has undergone dramatic evolution over the past several years. The application of radiofrequency ablation techniques to these arrhythmias has, in many cases, replaced medical therapy as the preferred therapeutic modality (Table 8.1). This, of course, has expanded the role of diagnostic studies in evaluation of these rhythms, and in turn greatly enhanced our understanding of the basic mechanisms underlying them.

The primary diagnostic tool for evaluating supraventricular arrhythmias remains the 12-lead ECG. In conjunction with vagal maneuvers or adenosine administration, the standard electrocardiogram can usually be used to identify the tachycardia mechanism. A simple approach is to identify the P wave and define its relationship to the QRS during tachycardia. This will place the arrhythmia into one of three categories: (A) long RP (atrial tachycardia, "atypical" AV nodal reentrant tachycardia, permanent form of junctional reentrant tachycardia, sinus node reentry, inappropriate sinus tachycardia); (B) short RP (atrial tachycardia, orthodromic atrioventricular tachycardia); and (C) typical AV nodal reentrant tachycardia in which the P wave is hidden in the QRS complex, or visible at the most terminal aspect of it.

Radiofrequency Ablation of Supraventricular Tachycardias

Ablation of the AV junction was first utilized in humans to treat supraventricular tachycardias with rapid ventricular response refractory to drug therapy.[13] A direct-current energy source was used, which was effective but barotrauma created large lesions in the myocardium. Currently, radiofrequency energy is used to produce small, controllable tissue lesions by heat. Advances in catheter design allow fine manipulation of the tip, further expanding the role of ablation to a variety of supraventricular and ventricular arrhythmias. Radiofrequency (RF) ablation is now considered primary therapy for a number of clinical situations, and has supplanted the role of cardiac surgery in these disorders. Recently, the U.S. ablation experience from 1989–1993 has been published as a survey by the North American Society of Pacing and Electrophysiology (NASPE).[14] This data documents the growth and success of ablation procedures over this time period (Figures 8.1 and 8.2).

Atrioventricular Reentrant Tachycardia

Atrioventricular reentrant tachycardia (AVRT), or Wolff-Parkinson-White syndrome, occurs as the result of a macro reentrant circuit that includes the AV node, ventric-

TABLE 8.1. Ablation Procedures Compared to Alternative Treatment Options for Supraventricular Tachyarrhythmias

SVT Type	Treatment Options	Estimated Success Rate	Complications*
Atrioventricular reentry (Wolff-Parkinson-White syndrome)	Beta blocker/ Calcium channel blocker	<50%	Bradycardia, AV block
	Antiarrhythmic drug	75–90%	Proarrhythmia, drug-specific side effects
	Ablation	90–95%	
AV nodal reentry	Beta blocker/ Calcium channel blocker	<50%	Bradycardia, AV block
	Antiarrhythmic drug	75–90%	Proarrhythmia, drug-specific side effects
	Ablation	97%	AV block
Atrial tachycardia	Antiarrhythmic drug	33%	Proarrhythmia, drug-specific side effects
	Ablation	90%	
Inappropriate sinus tachycardia	Beta blocker/ Calcium channel blocker	25%	Bradycardia, AV block
	Ablation	80–90%	Total nodal ablation
Atrial flutter	Antiarrhythmic drug	30%	Proarrhythmia, drug-specific side effects
	Ablation	85%	
Atrial fibrillation	Antiarrhythmic drug	50–75%	Proarrhythmia, drug-specific side effects
	Ablation (1) AV node (2) Atrial	97% Investigational	

*Ablation procedures including left heart catheterization incur the possible risks of damage to the aortic valve, coronary arteries, and pericardial tamponade. Significant complications in left-sided ablations occur in approximately 2%.

ular myocardium, and a myocardial bridge (accessory pathway) across the AV groove. Conduction through the circuit usually proceeds in an antegrade fashion down the AV node, through ventricular myocardium, and then in a retrograde direction over the AP (orthodromic tachycardia). This results in a narrow QRS complex tachycardia, in contrast to the preexcited wide QRS complex tachycardia (antidromic tachycardia) that results from antegrade conduction over the accessory pathway. Ablation is now considered the treatment of choice in most patients who

Naspe Survey on Catheter Ablation
No. of Procedures Performed in USA 1989-1993

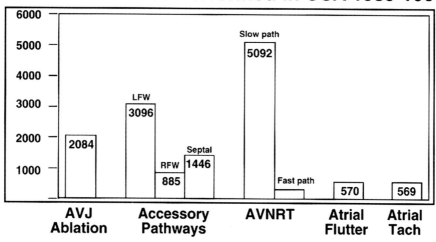

Figure 8.1. AVJ, atrioventricular junction; AVNRT, AV nodal reentry tachycardia; LFW, left free wall pathway; RFW, right free wall pathway; Sept, septal pathway. (From Scheinman, MM: NASPE Policy Statement: NASPE Survey on Catheter Ablation. PACE 1995 (18):1474)

Naspe Survey on Catheter Ablation
% Success 1989-1993

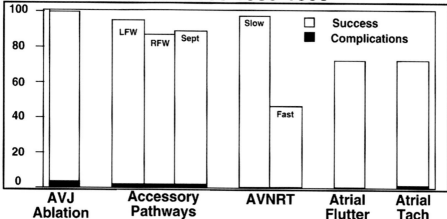

Figure 8.2. *AVJ*, atrioventricular junction; *AVNRT*, AV nodal reentrant tachycardia; *LFW*, left free wall pathway; *RFW*, right free wall pathway; *Sept*, septal pathway. (From Scheinman, MM: NASPE Policy Statement: NASPE Survey on Catheter Ablation. PACE 1995 (18):1474)

have symptomatic AV reentrant tachycardia, or atrial fibrillation with a rapid ventricular response due to conduction over the accessory pathway. The procedure is
safe, but not without risk. Of 3,981 AVRT ablations reported in the NASPE survey,
there were a total of 99 significant complications (2%). The most frequent major
adverse events included pericarditis (10 patients) and frank tamponade (7 patients).
Inadvertent AV block was reported in 9 patients, and 8 patients suffered cerebrovascular accidents. There were four procedure-related deaths.

AV Nodal Reentrant Tachycardia

The AV node may contain two or more distinct pathways that conduct at different
rates, and have different refractory periods. The "fast" pathway has a short refractory period and most commonly forms the retrograde limb of the reentry circuit,
while the "slow" pathway has a relatively long refractory period and usually forms
the anterograde limb of the circuit. Thus the terms "slow-fast" for the typical form
of AV nodal reentrant tachycardia (AVNRT), and "fast-slow" for the atypical form.
Of critical importance to the success of ablation of AVNRT is the finding that the
atrial connections of the slow pathway are located posteriorly, relatively remote
from the compact node. A lesion placed between the coronary sinus and the inferior vena cava is used to eliminate slow pathway conduction. The risk of AV block
following the procedure is approximately 1%. Given the safety and efficacy of ablative therapy for AVNRT, it may be considered as a primary therapeutic modality. It
is particularly appropriate for patients with symptomatic sustained tachycardia that
is drug resistant, or those who are drug intolerant. Ablation is also appropriate for
the patient who simply does not desire long-term drug therapy.

Atrial Tachycardia

Atrial tachycardia is most commonly due to enhanced automaticity of an atrial focus,
often located near the crista terminalis, around the upper pulmonary veins, or at the
base of the atrial appendages. It usually presents in children or young adults, and is
a cause of tachycardia-induced cardiomyopathy. As this arrhythmia is generally
resistant to medical therapy, and RF is frequently curative, we now consider ablation
as first-line therapy for atrial tachycardia. The focus is identified during invasive study
with "activation mapping," identifying the area of earliest local electrical activity relative to the surface P wave.[15] While technically challenging, ablation can be performed quite successfully (85–95% success rates) in centers that are experienced
with this procedure. As a large proportion of atrial tachycardia foci are located in
the left atrium, transseptal mapping and ablation is frequently required. Although
complication rates are low, there is increased risk of cardiac tamponade, systemic
embolization, and bleeding risk resulting from anticoagulation used in all left-sided
procedures.

Atrial Flutter

Endocardial mapping of atrial flutter has defined the mechanism of this arrhythmia
as a macro reentrant circuit, which, in its most common form travels in a counter-
clockwise direction in the right atrium. A zone of slow conduction of the circuit has

been found to lie on the floor of the right atrium, between the tricuspid annulus and the inferior vena cava. When RF lesions are placed across this "isthmus," flutter is reliably eliminated with success rates upwards of 85%. In our center, recurrence rates for atrial flutter are on the order of 5%. Approximately 10% may develop late atrial fibrillation. We now consider RF ablation to be a primary therapeutic modality in this rhythm, which is often difficult to control pharmacologically.

Atrial Fibrillation

Atrial fibrillation (AF) is the most common supraventricular arrhythmia, with an incidence of approximately 4% in the population over 60 yr of age. Drug therapy is usually ineffective in maintenance of sinus rhythm and is frequently associated with adverse effects. Ablation of the AV junction to control ventricular rates is commonly used in patients with AF who are refractory to or do not tolerate pharmacologic therapy. These patients require chronic pacemaker therapy.

Recent advances in treatment of atrial fibrillation associated with rapid ventricular response have been made by "modification" of the AV node. This procedure employs RF ablation in the region of the slow pathway approaches to the AV node, thereby eliminating that aspect of the node with the shortest refractory period. Significant decreases in ventricular rate have been achieved, but the long-term clinical value of this approach is yet to be defined.

An exciting area of clinical investigation is the use of RF ablation to eliminate atrial fibrillation. Akin to the "maze" procedure which surgically divides the atrial myocardium, placement of several long linear lesions in the atria have been shown to successfully eliminate atrial fibrillation in a small series of patients. A major limitation is the exceedingly long procedure time (12–18 hr), and the risk of cerebrovascular accident. New ablation catheters which create long linear lesions are in development, and promise to significantly expand the role of ablation in the therapy of this arrhythmia.

Inappropriate Sinus Tachycardia

This relatively uncommon but often debilitating arrhythmia may now be treated with RF modification of the sinus node. Successful application of RF energy has been facilitated by the use of intracardiac echocardiography (ICE), allowing anatomic localization of the sinus node by defining the superior vena caval–right atrial junction, and the crista terminalis. Lesions placed at the superior aspect of the crista terminalis reduce the sinus rate, presumably by eliminating the more rapid pacemaker cells and allowing for the emergence of a slower, more inferiorly placed pacemaker. Damage to the node can result in the need for permanent pacing, and thus this risk must be weighed against the benefits of ablative therapy.

Ventricular Tachyarrhythmias

The clinical approach to ventricular arrhythmias has evolved substantially over the past several years with the advent of the implantable cardioverter defibrillator (ICD), and mounting evidence that traditional antiarrhythmic therapy may not confer a sur-

TABLE 8.2. Ablation Procedures Compared to Alternative Treatment Options
for Ventricular Tachyarrhythmias

Ventricular Tachycardia Type	Treatment Options	Estimated Success Rate	Complications
RV outflow tract	Beta blocker/ Verapamil	60%	Bradycardia, AV block
	Antiarrhythmic drug	66%	Proarrhythmia, drug-specific side effects
	Ablation	90%	RV perforation
Left septal	Beta blocker/ Verapamil	50–70%	Bradycardia, AV block
	Antiarrhythmic drug	66%	Proarrhythmia, drug-specific side effects
	Ablation	85%	CVA, tamponade, arterial injury
Bundle-branch reentry	Ablation	100%	AV block requiring pacemaker
Ischemic or idiopathic dilated cardiomyopathy	Antiarrhythmic drugs (1) Noninducible (2) Inducible	65–100% 10–60%	Proarrhythmia, drug-specific side effects
	ICD	50%	Infection, pneumothorax, hematoma
	Ablation	60–70%	CVA, tamponade, arterial injury

Abbreviations: AV = atrioventricular; RV = right ventricular; CVA = cardiovascular accident; ICD = implantable cardioverter defibrillator.

vival benefit. Radiofrequency ablation has become a primary modality in the treatment of several uncommon forms of ventricular tachycardia (VT), but remains a less successful adjunct in the treatment of VT due to coronary artery disease (Table 8.2).

Nonsustained Ventricular Tachycardia

The risk of sudden cardiac death in patients having nonsustained ventricular tachycardia (NSVT) is dependent on underlying cardiac pathology. Patients with documented NSVT should have a thorough evaluation for structural or ischemic heart disease, which, if not found, defines a population at very low risk for future events. Therapy or invasive study is not necessary in these patients. However, patients with structural heart disease should be classified according to etiology, as the approach to treatment varies.

The most common clinical setting for NSVT is in the patient with coronary artery disease. Nonsustained VT frequently occurs in the first 48 hr postinfarction, and when present does not indicate a worse prognosis. However, when NSVT occurs past this time period, the risk of sudden death increases substantially, particularly in patients with depressed ejection fraction.[16,17]

Attempts have been made to further stratify these patients for risk of sudden cardiac death (SCD). Several studies have investigated the relationship between NSVT and other proven risk factors for arrhythmic events, such as signal-averaged ECG and inducible monomorphic ventricular tachycardia during invasive testing. A high-risk group may be defined on the basis of NSVT, a positive signal-averaged ECG, and poor ejection fraction. Studies have shown that these patients have a very high risk (50%) of developing VT or sudden cardiac death. Gomes and associates evaluated the value of programmed electrical stimulation in patients with high-grade premature ventricular contractions (PVCs) and no evidence of sustained VT, cardiac arrest, or syncope.[18] Their prospective study showed a higher incidence of cardiac events in patients with inducible VT (31.5%) compared to noninducible patients (7.8%). Wilber and associates studied 100 consecutive patients with spontaneous asymptomatic NSVT and ejection fraction less than 40%.[19] During follow-up of 16.7 months, the 1- and 2-yr incidence of cardiac arrest or sudden death was 2% and 6% in patients without inducible sustained ventricular arrhythmias, 0% and 11% in patients in whom inducible arrhythmias were suppressed with drug therapy, and 34% and 50% in patients with persistent inducible ventricular arrhythmias.

Therefore, a reasonable approach to the postmyocardial infarction patient with NSVT is to first evaluate the ejection fraction and signal-averaged ECG. Those who have an ejection fraction <40% and positive late potentials represent a high-risk group, who should then undergo invasive electrophysiologic studies. Patients with inducible ventricular arrhythmias may be treated with empiric amiodarone, guided antiarrhythmic medication, or ICD implantation. A number of prospective studies have been initiated to determine the preferable approach for these patients.

The incidence of NSVT in patients with idiopathic dilated cardiomyopathy varies between 20% and 60%, and most studies have found this to be a strong risk factor for sudden cardiac death.[20,21,22] In contrast to patients with coronary artery disease, however, investigators have been unable to further stratify these patients with invasive testing. A review of the studies evaluating the significance of inducible sustained monomorphic ventricular tachycardia in this population found that inducibility is associated with an increased risk of sudden death, but its absence did not define a low-risk group.[23–25] Therefore, negative studies may be misleading, and (apart from patients with bundle-branch reentrant-VT—see below) at this point there appears to be no value to invasive testing in these patients.

Sustained Ventricular Tachycardia and Cardiac Arrest

Reentry appears to be the dominant mechanism of sustained ventricular tachycardia in patients with ischemic cardiac disease. This arrhythmia can be triggered with programmed electrical stimulation to reproduce clinical arrhythmias in over 90% of patients with myocardial damage and documented sustained monomorphic VT. While rates of VT induction are lower in patients who present with either cardiac arrest or other forms of cardiomyopathy, early observational studies generated enthusiasm for using invasive testing to guide antiarrhythmic drug therapy.[26,27] There appeared to be a clear arrhythmia-free survival benefit in those patients with inducible VT at baseline, which, after administration of a drug, was rendered non-inducible at follow-up study. Even in those patients in whom VT remained inducible on drug, reduction of the VT cycle length by 100 msec or more (with hemodynamic stability) conferred the same mortality benefit.[28]

For several years this data directed the approach to treating patients with VT. It is not clear, however, whether arrhythmia-free survival was due to drug effect, or whether noninducibility on drug therapy simply selected patients at lower risk. It must also be emphasized that the substrate of the arrhythmia is not static, and is subject to variability based on several factors, including conditions of ischemia, catecholamine levels, electrolyte balance, and neurohumoral input. Therefore, while invasive testing may identify a drug in the laboratory which alters the substrate and renders it noninducible, it is difficult to predict whether an altered physiologic milieu over the course of time will render the drug ineffective. Similarly, invasive studies cannot be expected to detect the potential for proarrhythmic effects of drug treatment, a growing concern in the aftermath of the Cardiac Arrhythmia Suppression Trials (CAST).[29,30] On the other hand, failure to induce sustained ventricular tachycardia may not implicate the absence of an arrhythmogenic substrate.

Survivors of Cardiac Arrest

Survivors of cardiac arrest not associated with Q-wave infarction are at high risk for recurrent arrhythmias and sudden death. Mortality in this population is reported to be 24–30% at 1 yr, 34–40% at 2 yr, and 51–60% at 4 yr, with the cause of death usually recurrence of an initial arrhythmia (this compared to adjusted mortality of 20% at 4 yr in the general population).[31] These figures may be declining due to advances in therapy, and an overall decline in cardiac mortality, but these patients clearly remain at high risk.

As invasive testing is capable of identifying both tachycardic and bradycardic substrates, it is considered a standard diagnostic tool in this population. When studied in the baseline state (without antiarrhythmic therapy), up to 80% are found to have inducible VT. Approximately 40–50% of these tachycardias are sustained, monomorphic VT, with the remainder polymorphic VT, ventricular fibrillation (VF), or NSVT.[32–35] Successful suppression of sustained monomorphic VT with either drug or surgical therapy has been associated with an improved outcome, while patients discharged with inducible VT have a twofold risk of recurrent cardiac arrest. Unfortunately, VT is suppressible in only a minority of these patients.

Several recently published studies and ongoing trials will further define therapy in these patients, and the indications for invasive testing. The Cardiac Arrest in Seattle Conventional Versus Amiodarone Drug Evaluation (CASCADE) compared empirical amiodarone therapy versus conventional management guided either invasively or by Holter monitoring in survivors of out of hospital VF.[36] Patients treated with amiodarone had a lower recurrence rate of sudden cardiac death, resuscitated VF, and syncopal defibrillator shock. The conclusion that amiodarone therapy was superior was marred by its considerably higher incidence of serious side effects. The Amiodarone Versus Implantable Device (AVID), Canadian Implantable Device Study (CIDS), and Cardiac Arrest Study Hamburg (CASH) trials are in progress, comparing defibrillator and drug therapy in survivors of cardiac arrest or syncopal ventricular tachycardia.

Evaluation of Pharmacotherapy

The use of invasive studies in the assessment of antiarrhythmic drug therapy has developed from the observation that, in a large proportion of patients with inducible VT, a drug can be identified which renders the circuit noninducible with programmed stimulation.[37,38] These findings led to widespread use of invasive testing to guide antiarrhythmic therapy. However, drug therapy may also be guided noninvasively, through the use of Holter monitoring to document arrhythmia suppression. With either approach, patients receiving effective therapy have better outcomes than those with ineffective therapy. Recent clinical trials have compared the utility of these methods.

A Canadian trial and the Electrophysiologic Study Versus Electrocardiographic Monitoring (ESVEM) trial randomly evaluated the value of invasive versus noninvasive testing of drug efficacy for ventricular arrhythmias.[39,40] The Canadian trial found that in 57 patients with sustained VT the risk of recurrent ventricular tachycardia, ventricular fibrillation, or cardiac arrest after 2 yr was 43% in patients treated with drugs selected by the noninvasive approach. This figure compared to a 7% recurrence rate in patients treated with invasive guidance. The ESVEM trial, on the other hand, reached a different conclusion. In this study of 486 patients, the incidence of sudden death or arrhythmia recurrence was the same with either approach. Since very different protocols were used in these studies, the value of invasive testing to choose specific drug therapy is still a matter of debate.

Implantable Devices in the Treatment of Sustained Ventricular Tachycardia

Presently available ICDs provide the physician with a great deal of flexibility in the therapy of ventricular arrhythmias. These devices are capable of so-called tiered therapy, consisting of (1) antitachycardia pacing (ATP), (2) low-energy cardioversion, and (3) high-energy cardioversion. These choices place greater emphasis on the predischarge invasive study, which is used to test and optimally program the device.

Antitachycardia pacing provides a painless option in patients with monomorphic, sustained, hemodynamically stable VT. Unfortunately, a complication of this mode of therapy is acceleration of the VT to a more rapid monomorphic tachycardia, polymorphic VT, or VF requiring defibrillation. The efficacy and safety of ATP must be tested in the electrophysiology laboratory prior to patient discharge. Low-energy cardioversion is an alternative approach used for patients with monomorphic, hemodynamically stable VT that saves energy and in most cases is less painful than that reported with high-energy shocks. Similar to ATP, low-energy cardioversion carries the risk of VT acceleration or VF, and therefore must also be tested in the electrophysiology laboratory prior to its use.

Catheter Ablation in the Treatment of Sustained Ventricular Tachycardia

Patients with monomorphic VT may be candidates for RF ablation. The use of this therapy requires the presence of an inducible, hemodynamically stable ventricular arrhythmia and the ability to localize the reentrant circuit or automatic focus with endocardial mapping. The outcome of ablation has varied depending on the patient population, as outlined below.

Bundle-branch Reentry Ventricular Tachycardia

Bundle-branch reentry ventricular tachycardia (BBR-VT) has a reported incidence of 6% among patients with sustained monomorphic VTs.[41] This arrhythmia is most commonly found in patients with idiopathic dilated cardiomyopathy. The predominant clinical presentation is syncope or sudden cardiac death. The circuit is well defined and composed of the right and left bundle branches and the transseptal myocardial tissue. Catheter ablation of the right bundle branch is a simple procedure and provides a permanent cure, and thus is considered primary therapy in these patients. On follow-up, the incidence of sudden cardiac death or requirement of a permanent pacemaker is low. However, associated VT of myocardial origin is an important complicating factor.

Idiopathic Ventricular Tachycardia

Ventricular tachycardia may occur in patients without structural heart disease. These arrhythmias usually originate from the right ventricular outflow tract, and have a left bundle branch/inferior axis morphology, or from the infero-apical area of the left ventricular septum with resultant right bundle branch block/superior axis morphology.

Right ventricular outflow tract VT is seen in young to middle-aged subjects, is most often of the repetitive monomorphic type and is generally not associated with symptoms. In contrast, paroxysmal VT, often precipitated by exercise, may be associated with severe symptoms. This rhythm is usually not inducible with programmed stimulation, but requires administration of atrial or ventricular overdrive pacing. It may be controlled with beta blockers and calcium channel blockers, particularly if the arrhythmia is provoked by exercise.

Idiopathic left septal VT is most common in young patients. Although syncope and hemodynamic collapse are rare, patients are often symptomatic with sustained episodes of tachycardia. This rhythm can usually be induced and terminated with programmed stimulation, and is usually responsive to verapamil.

As the majority of patients with idiopathic VT are young, and there is the possibility of a permanent cure eliminating the need for medications, catheter ablation procedures are being increasingly used in this population with high success rates in experienced centers.

Ischemic Ventricular Tachycardia

In comparison to the experience with BBR-VT and idiopathic ventricular tachycardia, ablation in the setting of an ischemic substrate has been less successful. Endocardial mapping of the circuit is more problematic, and the risk of the procedure is certainly higher in this population. The majority of patients still require at least one additional mode of therapy following the procedure. For these reasons, the role of RF at this time is generally as an adjunct to device or drug therapy.

In summary, there are several options available in the treatment of the patient with sustained VT, including: (1) antiarrhythmic therapy guided either by a noninvasive or invasive approach, (2) empiric amiodarone therapy, (3) radiofrequency catheter ablation, and (4) ICD implantation. The outcome of several ongoing clinical trials will serve to clarify the issue of which approach is optimal. The authors' approach to the patient with new onset sustained ventricular tachycardia includes invasive electrophysiologic testing. The importance of the initial study lies in the ability to establish the diagnosis and to exclude treatable forms of tachycardia, such as bundle-branch reentry–VT, variants of Wolff-Parkinson-White syndrome (WPW) (i.e., Mahaim tracts), or other forms of paroxysmal supraventricular tachycardia. A trial of drug therapy with amiodarone or sotalol is then initiated and assessed with a follow-up electrophysiologic study. Patients who fail drug therapy are then managed with ICDs, occasionally with an adjunctive antiarrhythmic agent.

Syncope

Syncope is a dramatic and commonly encountered symptom which demands thorough evaluation to establish its etiology. The advent of head-up tilt testing has helped identify the neurocardiogenic mechanism, which is now recognized as the most common cause in patients without structural heart disease. However, in patients with manifest cardiac disease, or with significant risk factors, syncope often heralds a life-threatening underlying tachyarrhythmia or bradyarrhythmia requiring specific diagnosis. The 1-yr mortality in patients with a cardiovascular cause of syncope is reported to be 18–33%, compared with 0–12% in patients with syncope with a noncardiovascular cause, or syncope of unknown origin.[42–44]

The use of invasive study in the evaluation of syncopal patients is driven by the necessity to evaluate risk for sudden cardiac death. While clues to the etiology of syncope may be gleaned from ambulatory monitoring, echocardiography, and the 12-lead ECG, their yield is too low to establish a definitive diagnosis in most cases. Additionally, several studies have observed a dissociation between syncope recurrence and sudden death risk, suggesting that the mechanisms may be different.[43,45,46] Invasive testing allows identification of previously undiagnosed sinus node disease, conduction block, supraventricular and ventricular arrhythmias. Clearly, patients with underlying cardiac pathology represent a subgroup at highest risk for these abnormalities that requires aggressive evaluation soon after presentation.

We study all patients with structural heart disease and syncope that is unexplained after initial noninvasive testing. Further, patients without structural heart disease but who have recurrent syncope and negative tilt test are invasively evaluated.

CONCLUSION

This chapter has emphasized the indications for invasive electrophysiologic studies, with particular attention to their impact on therapeutic decisions. The authors have presented their approach, but it must be emphasized that the application of these procedures requires clinical judgment, and decisions are tailored to the individual patient. It should also be evident that these indications are evolving, largely due to the development of safe and effective radiofrequency ablation. RF has significantly altered the approach to most supraventricular arrhythmias as it has become a primary therapeutic modality, replacing often poorly tolerated or ineffective pharmacologic choices. The development of successful ablation procedures for some ventricular arrhythmias has also underscored the necessity of invasive studies in the evaluation of these patients. In the future the indications for invasive studies are likely to broaden, as rapid advances in catheter and mapping technology allow successful ablation therapy of such common arrhythmias as atrial fibrillation and ventricular tachycardia in the setting of coronary artery disease.

REFERENCES

1. Scherlag BJ, Lau SH, Helfant RA, et al: Catheter technique for recording His bundle stimulation and recording in the intact dog. *J Appl Physiol* 25:425, 1968.
2. Durrer D, Schoo L, Schuilenburg RM, et al: The role of premature beats in the initiation and termination of supraventricular tachycardias in the WPW syndrome. *Circulation* 36: 644, 1967.
3. Coumel P, Cabrol C, Fabiato A, et al: Tachycardiamente par rythme reciproque. *Arch Mal Coeur* 60:1830, 1967.
4. Wellens HJJ: *Electrical Stimulation of the Heart in the Study and Treatment of Tachycardias.* Leiden, Stenfert Kroese, 1971.
5. Scheinman MM, Peters RW, Sauve MJ, et al: Value of the H-Q interval in patients with bundle branch block and the role of prophylactic permanent pacing. *Am J Cardiol* 50: 1316, 1982.
6. Zipes DP, DiMarco JP, Gillette PC, et al: Guidelines for clinical intracardiac electrophysiological and catheter ablation procedures: a report of the American College of Cardiology/American Heart Association Task Force on Practice Guidelines. *JACC* 26:555–573, 1995.
7. Rosen KM, Loeb HS, Sinno MZ, et al: Cardiac conduction in patients with symptomatic sinus node disease. *Circulation* 43:836, 1971.
8. Dhigra RA, Denes P, Wu D, et al: The significance of second degree atrioventricular block and bundle branch block: observations regarding site and type of block. *Circulation* 49:638–646, 1974.
9. McAnulty JH, Rahimtoola SH, Murphy E, et al: Natural history of "high risk" bundle branch block. *N Engl J Med* 307:137, 1982.
10. Rosen KM, Dhingra RC, Wyndham C: Significance of H-V intervalin 515 patients with chronic bifascicular block. *Am J Cardiol* 45:405, 1980.
11. Scheinman M, Peters R, Sauve M, et al: Value of the H-Q interval in patients with bundle branch block and the role of prophylactic permanent pacing. *Am J Cardiol* 50: 1316–1322, 1982.
12. Dhingra RC, Wyndham C, Baurnfeind R, et al: Significance of block distal to the His bundle induced by atrial pacing in patients with chronic bifascicular block. *Circulation* 60: 1455, 1979.
13. Scheinman M, Morady F, Hess D, et al: Catheter-induced ablation of the atrioventricular junction to control refractory supraventricular arrhythmias. *JAMA* 248:851–855, 1982.
14. Scheinman M: NASPE policy statement: NASPE survey on catheter ablation. *PACE* 18:1474–1478, 1995.
15. Lesh MD: Radiofrequency catheter ablation of atrial tachycardia and flutter. In Zipes DP,

Jalife: *Cardiac Electrophysiology: From Cell to Bedside*. Philadelphia, WB Saunders, 1994, pp 1461–1477.

16. Anderson KP, De Camilla J, Moss AJ, et al: Clinical significance of ventricular tachycardia (3 beats or longer) detected during ambulatory monitoring after myocardial infarction. *Circulation* 57:890–897, 1978.

17. Bigger JT, Weld FM, Rolnitzky LM: The prevalence and significance of ventricular tachycardia detected by ambulatory ECG recordings in the late phase of acute myocardial infarction. *Am J Cardiol* 48:815–821, 1981.

18. Gomes JC, Hariman RI, Kang PS, et al: Programmed electrical stimulation in patients with high-grade ventricular ectopy: electrophysiologic findings and prognosis for survival. *Circulation* 70:43–51, 1984.

19. Wilber DJ, Olshamsky B, Moran JF, et al: Electrophysiological testing and nonsustained ventricular tachycardia: use and limitations in patients with coronary artery disease and impaired ventricular function. *Circulation* 82:350–358, 1990.

20. Meinertz T, Hoffmann T, Kasper W, et al: Significance of ventricular arrhythmias in idiopathic dilated cardiomyopathy. *Am J Cardiol* 53:902–907, 1984.

21. Costanzo-Nordin MR, O'Connell JB, Engelmeier RS, et al: Ventricular tachycardia in dilated cardiomyopathy: a variable independent of hemodynamics, morphology, and prognosis. *J Am Coll Cardiol* 3:594, 1984.

22. Gradman A, Deedwania P, Cody R, et al: Predictors of sudden death in mild to moderate heart failure. *J Am Coll Cardiol* 14:564–570, 1989.

23. Gossinger HD, Jung M, Wagner L, et al: Prognostic role of inducible ventricular tachycardia in patients with dilated cardiomyopathy and asymptomatic nonsustained ventricular tachycardia. *Int J Cardiol* 29:215–220, 1990.

24. Meinertz T, Treese N, Kasper W, et al: Determinants of prognosis in idiopathic dilated cardiomyopathy as determined by programmed electrical stimulation. *Am J Cardiol* 56:337, 1985.

25. Brembilla-Perrot B, Donneti J, Terrier de la Chaise A, et al: Diagnostic value of ventricular stimulation in patients with idiopathic dilated cardiomyopathy. *Am Heart J* 121:1124–1131, 1991.

26. Wilber D, Garan H, Finkelstein D, et al: Out-of-hospital cardiac arrest: use of electrophysiologic testing in the prediction of long-term outcome. *N Engl J Med* 318:19–24, 1988.

27. Swerdlow CD, Winkle R, Mason J: Determinants of survival in patients with ventricular tachyarrhythmias. *N Engl J Med* 308:1436–1442, 1983.

28. Waller TJ, Kay HR, Spielman SR, et al: Reduction in sudden death and total mortality by antiarrhythmic therapy evaluated by electrophysiologic drug testing: criteria of efficacy in patients with sustained ventricular tachyarrhythmia. *J Am Coll Cardiol* 10:83–89, 1987.

29. The Cardiac Arrhythmia Suppression Trial (CAST) Investigators: Preliminary report: effect of encainide and flecainide on mortality in a randomized trial of arrhythmia suppression after myocardial infarction. *N Engl J Med* 321:406–410, 1989.

30. Cardiac Arrhythmia Suppression Trial Investigators: Effect of the antiarrhythmic agent moricizine on survival after myocardial infarction. *N Engl J Med* 327:227–233, 1992.

31. Eisenberg M, Hallstrom A, Bergner L: Long-term survival after out-of-hospital cardiac arrest. *N Engl J Med* 306:1340–1343, 1982.

32. Benditt DG, Benson DW, Klein GJ, et al: Prevention of recurrent sudden cardiac arrest: role of provocative electropharmacologic testing. *J Am Coll Cardiol* 2:418–425, 1983.

33. Morady F, Scheinman M, Hess D, et al: Electrophysiologic testing in the management of survivors of out-of-hospital cardiac arrest. *Am J Cardiol* 51:85–89, 1983.

34. Ruskin J, DiMarco J, Garan H: Out-of-hospital cardiac arrest: electrophysiologic observations and selection of long-term antiarrhythmic therapy. *N Engl J Med* 303:607–613, 1980.

35. Wilber D, Garan H, Finkelstein D, et al: Out-of-hospital cardiac arrest: use of electrophysiologic testing in the prediction of long-term outcome. *N Engl J Med* 318:19–24, 1988.

36. CASCADE investigators: Randomized antiarrhythmic drug therapy in survivors of cardiac arrest (the CASCADE study). *Am J Cardiol* 72:280–287, 1993.

37. Mason J, Winkle R: Electrode-catheter arrhythmia induction in the selection and assessment of antiarrhythmic drug therapy for recurrent ventricular tachycardia. *Circulation* 58:971–985, 1978.

38. Horowitz L, Josephson M, Farshidi A, et al: Recurrent sustained ventricular tachycardia. 3. Role of electrophysiologic study in selection of antiarrhythmic regimens. *Circulation* 58:986–997, 1978.

39. Mitchell LB, Duff HJ, Manyari DE, et al: A randomized clinical trial of the noninvasive and invasive approaches to drug therapy of ventricular tachycardia. *N Engl J Med* 317:1681–1687, 1987.

40. Mason JW: A randomized comparison of electrophysiologic study to electrocardiographic monitoring for prediction of antiarrhythmic drug efficacy in patients with ventricular tachyarrhythmias. *N Engl J Med* 329:452–458, 1993.

41. Caceres J, Jazayeri M, McKinnie J, et al: Sustained bundle branch reentry as a mechanism of clinical tachycardia. *Circulation* 79:256–270, 1988.

42. Day S, Cook E, Funkenstein H, et al: Evaluation and outcome of emergency room patients with transient loss of consciousness. *Am J Med* 73:15–23, 1982.

43. Kapoor WN: Evaluation and outcome of patients with syncope. *Medicine* 69:160–175, 1990.

44. Siverstein M, Singer D, Mulley A, et al: Patients with syncope admitted to medical intensive care units. *JAMA* 248:1185–1189, 1982.

45. Doherty JU, Pembrook-Rogers D, Grogan E, et al: Electrophysiologic evaluation and follow-up characteristics of patients with recurrent unexplained syncope and presyncope. *Am J Cardiol* 55:703–708, 1985.

46. Bass EB, Elson JJ, Fogoros R, et al: Long-term prognosis of patients undergoing electrophysiologic studies for syncope of unknown origin. *Am J Cardiol* 62:1186–1191, 1988.

— 9 —

Coronary Angiography

Neal S. Kleiman, M.D.
Albert E. Raizner, M.D.

Coronary angiography has rapidly become an established part of the armamentarium for the diagnosis of patients with coronary artery disease and suspected coronary artery disease. While once the purview of a few specialized centers, the technique has now become widely applicable due to improvement in the equipment used, increases in operator skill, and improvements in the management of patients who have undergone angiography. The growth in coronary angiography has come about through two mechanisms. First, as catheters have become smaller in diameter and contrast agents have become more refined, the risk associated with coronary angiography has dropped dramatically. Second, the widespread availability of coronary artery bypass surgery and percutaneous transluminal angioplasty have led to a need for angiographic information on an ever increasing number of patients.

DESCRIPTION OF TECHNIQUE

The actual techniques used for coronary arteriography have undergone little evolution since the procedure was first developed. Access to a major arterial branch is obtained, the diagnostic catheter is advanced through the arterial system into the ascending aorta, and the diagnostic catheter is then placed in the coronary sinuses. The coronary ostia are then cannulated selectively, and radiographic contrast medium is injected into each ostium. A consecutive series of projections are obtained of each coronary. After the desired angiograms have been made and adjunctive information (i.e., hemodynamic measurements and angiography of other structures) obtained, the catheter is removed and homeostasis obtained.

161

Femoral Artery Approach

The femoral artery approach is most commonly used because of the easy accessibility and large caliber of the femoral artery. After local analgesia is administered, a small skin incision is made with a surgical blade, the skin bluntly dilated with a hemostat, and the artery punctured with an 18-gauge needle. A guidewire is advanced through the needle and an arterial introducer sheath with a hemostatic diaphragm is placed in the artery. Catheters are then advanced up the iliac artery and the aorta over a guidewire to the aortic root. Catheters used for this purpose are generally 5 or 6 French in diameter. After completion of the procedure, local pressure is applied to the femoral artery until hemostasis is achieved. The patient is subsequently kept at strict bed rest for 4 to 6 hr and advised to avoid activities which may require sudden or forceful movement of the hip for 24–48 hr thereafter.

The femoral approach is also favored because it easily accommodates the large-bore catheters which are required for some interventional procedures and because it allows angiographic access to both subclavian arteries so that injection of both internal mammary arteries may be performed. Injection of the gastroepiploic artery can also be performed from this location if needed. Its disadvantages arise from the potential presence of atherosclerotic obstructive disease in the iliac arteries and thoracoabdominal aorta, as well as from the relatively deep location of the femoral artery. Because the femoral artery lies several centimeters below the skin and dives beneath the peritoneal lining just superior to the inguinal ligament, bleeding from it following an angiographic procedure can go unnoticed until a relatively large amount of blood has been lost in the retroperitoneum or femoral space. This sort of problem is most common in the elderly, the obese, and patients who are vigorously anticoagulated.

Brachial Artery Approach

Initially, the brachial artery approach was widely used for coronary arteriography but it has become much less often utilized than the femoral approach. Its advantage lies in the easy accessibility of the brachial artery which in most individuals lies 1 or 2 cm below the surface of the skin. The approach also avoids the difficulties associated with disease in the iliac arteries and abdominal aorta, although tortuosity of the brachial vessels can make this approach difficult as well.

As originally developed, the brachial approach was performed using a surgical cutdown to and incision of the brachial artery. Generally, a woven dacron (Sones) catheter is used when this approach is selected; however, an introducer sheath and catheter can also be used. Following arteriographic and hemodynamic studies, the catheter is removed, antegrade and retrograde flow from the brachial artery ascertained, and the vessel repaired using one of a number of surgical closure techniques. More recently, percutaneous puncture of the brachial artery under local analgesia without surgical exposure of the vessel has become popular.

The advantage of the brachial approach is that it does not require the prolonged period of limited mobility required after femoral arterial puncture. On the other hand, motion of the arm is restricted for 24 hr. A major limitation of this technique is that in some patients, particularly women, the brachial artery is of a caliber too small to allow unimpeded passage of the catheter. In addition, entry of the angiographic catheter into the subclavian artery, usually for purposes of selective injection into the internal mammary artery, is limited to the ipsilateral side. Radiation exposure to the operator is considerably higher when the brachial approach is used. Serious hemorrhage is extremely rare when the brachial approach is used, however, local occlusion of the brachial artery due to either thrombosis or a dissection flap occurs more commonly.

Radial Artery Approach

This approach has found occasional use in recent years. The radial artery is cannulated with a needle which is subsequently exchanged for a 5 or 6 French sheath. Preformed catheters can be used when this approach is selected. From the operator's perspective, radial artery catheterization shares some similarities to the femoral approach since the wrist can be placed in the same vicinity as the patient's groin. Its obvious advantage is that patient mobility after the procedure is not limited. However, it does require that the radial artery be of relatively large caliber and that an ulnar artery supply flow to the hand. An Allen test should always be performed prior to performing radial artery catheterization.

DEVELOPMENTAL PERSPECTIVES

While postmortem angiography of the coronary arteries has been performed by pathologists since 1900, coronary angiography in (living) patients has been in use only for the last 35 yr and has been in widespread use for the last 20 yr. Selective coronary angiography owes its discovery to a fortuitous accident which beset Dr. Mason Sones in 1959, during which an angiographic catheter inadvertently entered a coronary artery during dye injection.[1] The coronary circulation was beautifully opacified and the patient suffered no ill consequences.

At approximately the same time, coronary artery physiologic experiments by Gregg[2] and later by Gould et al.[3] led to the application of fluid dynamic principles to the coronary circulation. The recognition that narrowing of a coronary artery lumen by more than 70% limited flow through the vessel and impaired vasodilator reserve in the distal coronary bed provided physiologic significance to angiographic findings. A new era was introduced with the observation that the extent of coronary artery disease, expressed as the number of major coronary arteries with significant luminal narrowing, as well as the ejection fraction determined by left ventricular angiography, was a powerful predictor of a patient's prognosis.[4,5] Further, the widespread use of coronary angiography in the late 1960s ultimately led to a new gold standard for the diagnosis of coronary artery disease. When subjected to coronary angiography, many patients who were previously thought to have disabling or unstable angina did not have coronary artery disease at all. These findings thus highlight the limitations of the clinical history and the electrocardiogram for diagnosing coronary artery disease.

TECHNICAL CONSIDERATIONS

Contrast Medium

The toxicity of radiocontrast medium constitutes the primary limitation of coronary arteriography. A variety of contrast agents is now available. Contrast agents are generally grouped according to their ionic or nonionic nature and their osmolality. The first generations of contrast agents were ionic, high osmolar compounds. Later generations were considerably lower in ionic content and osmolality but were also much more expensive. Injection of contrast medium into the circulation induces a variety of physiologic changes including activation of platelets,[6] alterations in the cross-linking of fibrinogen,[7] depression of myocardial contractility,[8] and alterations in renal blood flow. Ionic agents cause more depression of myocardial contractility and bradycardia on direct injection into the coronary circulation,[8] but less platelet activation.[6] As a result, use of nonionic normo-osmolar contrast agents is recommended in patients who are hemodynamically unstable, but the selection of specific agents in more stable patients is a matter of controversy, primarily due to economic issues.

The principal toxicity of radiocontrast administration is renal insufficiency. The mechanism of this toxicity is not clearly defined. Patients at greatest risk for contrast-induced nephrotoxicity are those with underlying renal insufficiency, diabetics, and the elderly. The risk is also increased in patients who are volume depleted and in those who have congestive heart failure. In prospective series, the incidence of an increase in serum creatinine has been reported to be as high as 37%[9] in diabetic patients with underlying azotemia. In another prospective series, Solomon reported that 26% of patients with mild to moderate renal insufficiency (baseline serum creatinine >1.6 mg/dl, mean 2.1 mg/dl) who underwent coronary arteriography had rises in serum creatinine exceeding 0.5 mg/dl.[10] The serum creatinine usually reaches a peak on the fourth day and declines to normal in 7 to 10 days. Serious sequelae are uncommon, although dialysis is occasionally required, and, in patients with severe underlying renal insufficiency, the loss of glomerular function can be permanent. Thus, the decision to undertake angiography in patients with preexistent renal insufficiency should take into account the likelihood that the need for chronic hemodialysis will be accelerated by the procedure. Minimizing the amount of contrast used, preprocedure volume expansion and the use of calcium channel blockers lessen the likelihood of developing contrast nephropathy.

INDICATIONS AND USES

The indications for coronary arteriography are undergoing constant change. Perhaps the most clearly stated indication for coronary arteriography is also the least meaningful; that is, when there is a need to know the patient's coronary anatomy. Even this broad objective must be undertaken with the understanding that coronary angiography yields, at best, a limited approximation of the status of the coronary arterial circulation. Multiple pathologic studies have demonstrated that because angiography displays a two-dimensional outline of the coronary arterial lumen, it underestimates the amount of atherosclerosis present, largely because of the diffuse nature of the disease[11,12] (Figure 9.1). Comparisons between intracoronary ultrasound findings and angiography have also stressed this point and have highlighted the limited ability of the angiogram to detect lesser amounts of lumenal narrowing and to identify calcification within the arterial wall.[13,14] Observations that myocardial infarction occurs as a result of rupture of an atherosclerotic plaque that initially produces only limited lumenal compromise also stress the point that imaging of the arterial lumen is of limited help in predicting the likelihood of specific cardiac events. Intracoronary angioscopic studies have also pointed out the limited sensitivity of angiography to detect intracoronary thrombus. Furthermore, there is a large interobserver variability when coronary angiograms are interpreted,[15,16] although quantitative measurement techniques have reduced these variations.[17] Despite these limitations, coronary angiography has proven very useful in delineating the anatomic correlates of specific problems (i.e., identifying the atheroma responsible for a myocardial infarction or the anatomic substrate responsible for an episode of unstable angina), and in planning the appropriate course of action. Perhaps equally important, the identification of patients with normal or minimal coronary artery disease who have a low likelihood of subsequent coronary events,[18,19] as well as those with severe multivessel disease whose likelihood of a coronary event is high, has withstood the test of time and contributed to the widespread use of angiography. The remainder of this chapter will describe the utility of coronary arteriography in a variety of clinical settings (Table 9.1).

Stable Angina

In patients with stable angina pectoris, the risk of myocardial infarction and cardiac death is low. Event rates in these patient groups have been best studied in the Coronary Artery Surgery Study (CASS) and Veterans Affairs (VA) cooperative trials during the 1970s. The medical management of patients with coronary artery disease has undergone a variety of changes over the last two decades. Unfortunately, prognostic data for medically managed patients, for the most part, were accrued during the 1970s. In the CASS trial, infarct-free survival for medically managed patients with stable angina pectoris and three-vessel disease was 83% at 5 yr, while that for patients with three-vessel disease was 77%. In patients with reduced ejection fractions, infarct-free survival rates were 72% and 63%, respectively. In patients with good left ventricular function (ejection fraction > 0.50), these rates were not different between patients treated medically or surgically.[20] In a more recent study of percutaneous transluminal coronary angioplasty (PTCA) versus medical therapy in patients with stable angina, over a 6-month period, the rate of myocardial infarction among medically treated patients with single-vessel disease was only 3%, whereas 46% became free of angina while on medical therapy.[21] Consequently, the need for coronary arteriography in patients with stable angina and preserved ventricular function is in large part predicated by the patient's symptomatic status rather than the need to improve prognosis.

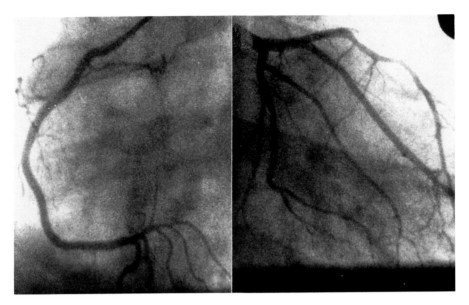

A

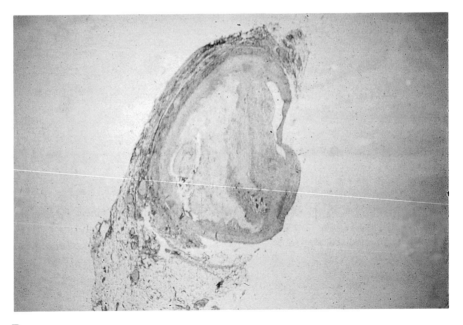

B

Figure 9.1. The limitations of coronary angiography are dramatically illustrated in this patient. (A) Only "minor" luminal irregularities are seen in the right and left coronary arteriograms performed several weeks before the patient's demise. (B) Histologic section at autopsy revealed extensive atherosclerosis obliterating most of the true original lumen. The remaining lumen (*right side of section*) represents only a small portion of the original lumen.

TABLE 9.1. Indications For Coronary Angiography

1. Stable angina
    Function-limiting symptoms
    Objective evidence of major ischemia
    Repetitive silent ischemia
2. Unstable angina
    Postmyocardial infarction
    Class IIb or IIIb unstable angina
    Class I unstable angina with:
       ischemia at low workloads
       large amount of myocardium at risk
3. Myocardial infarction
    Prelude to "direct" or "primary" PTCA
    Recurrent ischemia
    Ischemic response on stress test
    Patients with mechanical complications
       (Ventricular septal defect [VSD], mitral valve dysfunction)
4. Angioplasty follow-up
    Recurrent ischemia post-PTCA
    High-risk lesions
5. Peripheral vascular disease undergoing
    Surgery
    Demonstrable ischemia on stress test
    Symptomatic angina
    Ascending aortic aneurysm surgery
6. Noncoronary cardiac surgery
    Adults undergoing valve surgery
    Complex congenital heart disease
7. Congestive heart failure
    High risk factor profile
    Over 40 yr of age
    ECG evidence of prior infarction
    Angina or provocable ischemia
    Heart transplantation

Need for Triage

On the other hand, the need for more precise methods of triage and prognostication has led to more specific categorization of patients with stable angina for whom coronary arteriography is indicated. Detection of patients with symptoms of angina pectoris but who have angiographically normal coronary arteries identifies a group of patients in whom the likelihood of a catastrophic cardiac event is low and who often can be withdrawn from antianginal therapy, thereby sparing them from troublesome side effects.[18] However, it is increasingly appreciated that many episodes of ischemia are asymptomatic and that in some patients most of these episodes are "silent". The latter discovery would imply that medical control of anginal symptoms may be inadequate if ischemic episodes are not eliminated or reduced. Although this hypothesis has not been formally tested in an adequate sample of patients, the results of at least one randomized pilot study indicate that in patients with asymptomatic ischemia, survival at one year is increased by revascularization compared with suppression of ischemia using a combination of a beta blocker and calcium channel entry blocker.[22] The development of quantitative nuclear scintigraphic techniques has been shown by several groups of investigators to permit stratification of patients into high- and low-risk categories based on the amount of myocardium that becomes ischemic during stress. Ischemic responses exceeding 15–20% of the myocardium are associated with decrements in survival.[23] In such patients coronary angiography is indicated with the intent of revascularization.

In other individuals, the indications for angiography are largely dependent on whether there is a pressing need for a precise diagnosis, e.g., patients who are employed in occupations that are potentially hazardous to themselves or to others, such as pilots and bus drivers. Similarly, the threshold for performing angiography should be lower in patients who are extremely physically active.

Unstable Angina

The term *unstable angina* has taken on an extremely broad meaning, involving patients with a wide variety of illnesses ranging from angina beginning within 3 months prior to presentation, to rest angina at the time of presentation, and including a variety of noncardiac causes. A classification recently introduced by Braunwald has clarified this issue considerably. This classification distinguishes patients with "secondary" unstable angina and those with postinfarction angina from patients with "primary" unstable angina. Among the latter, it distinguishes angina at rest or on exertion and those with rest angina within 24 hr, from those with more remote episodes[2,4] (Table 9.2). Differing prognoses among patients in these classes has sub-

TABLE 9.2. Classification of Unstable Angina

	Clinical Circumstances		
	A. Develops in presence of extracardiac condition that intensifies myocardial ischemia (secondary UA)	B. Develops in absence of extracardiac condition (primary UA)	C. Develops within 2 wk after acute myocardial infarction (postinfarction UA)
I. New onset of severe angina or accelerated angina; no rest pain	IA	IB	IC
II. Angina at rest within past month but not within preceding 48 hr (Angina at rest, subacute)	IIA	IIB	IIC
III. Angina at rest within 48 hr (Angina at rest, acute)	IIIA	IIIB	IIIC

sequently been validated.[25] "Primary" unstable angina in Braunwald classes IIB and IIIB is characterized in many cases by plaque rupture and a prothrombotic milieu within the coronary circulation. It would seem reasonable that angiography would be useful to identify the location of plaque rupture (Figure 9.2) and that revascularization would restore antegrade flow in the blood vessel thus avoiding the progression to complete occlusion. This hypothesis was tested in the Thrombolysis in Myocardial Ischemia Phase III (TIMI IIIB) study. In this study, 1,473 patients with unstable angina within 24 hr and either ST or T wave changes or a prior history of coronary artery disease were randomized to receive a low dose of tissue plasminogen activator (t-PA) or a placebo; they were subsequently randomized to undergo coronary angiography with anatomically directed revascularization at 18 to 48 hr or to undergo a noninvasive investigation consisting of exercise testing with thallium injection and Holter monitoring for recurrent ischemia. The primary endpoint was a composite at 42 days of death, myocardial (re)infarction, or refractory ischemia mandating repeat catheterization. No differences in the frequency of death or myocardial infarction were present at the 42-day point. However, 64% of patients randomized to the "early conservative" strategy had an event leading to angiography within the 6-wk time frame, and the majority of these procedures occurred prior to hospital discharge.[26] Thus, there appeared to be little or no advantage in attempting to avoid or delay angiography. In addition, patients managed with the "early conservative" strategy required more rehospitalizations, spent more days in the hospital, and required more antianginal medications during the 6-wk period. At the end of one year, there were still no differences in catastrophic events but patients managed with the "early conservative" strategy spent more days in the hospital.[27]

The indications for angiography in patients with unstable angina thus depend on what class of instability is present and what facilities for angiography are available. For patients in whom unstable angina is secondary to another etiology, correction of the underlying cause (i.e., anemia or thyrotoxicosis) is indicated, followed by noninvasive evaluation. For patients with unstable angina following a recent myocardial infarction, angiography should be performed. For patients who fit Braunwald classes IIb and IIIb, the situation is more flexible. If angiography is not desired by the patient, or if the facilities for cardiac catheterization are not readily available, then a strategy directed toward noninvasive evaluation is acceptable, provided that the patient remains clinically free of angina or congestive heart failure. Referral for angiography will thus depend on the outcome of the noninvasive studies; patients with provocative tests that reveal ischemia at low workloads, or in whom a large amount of myocardium appears to be at risk, will need invasive evaluation. Alternatively, if the clinical facility is capable of supporting a high volume of coronary angiography, patients with class IIb or IIIb unstable angina may undergo an invasive workup strategy directly without the need for noninvasive testing (Figure 9.3). This approach has the advantage that a "cooling off" period of several days is not required; angiography may be performed on the first or second day after admission. Two other advantages are that patients with minimal coronary artery disease who make up approximately 20% of patients with a diagnosis of unstable angina[28] are quickly identified and directed toward more fruitful areas of investigation, and patients with significant coronary artery disease are spared the necessity of having to undergo two sets of studies. Occasionally, patients with unstable angina are found to have coronary artery spasm (Figure 9.4). It is now quite clear that it is important

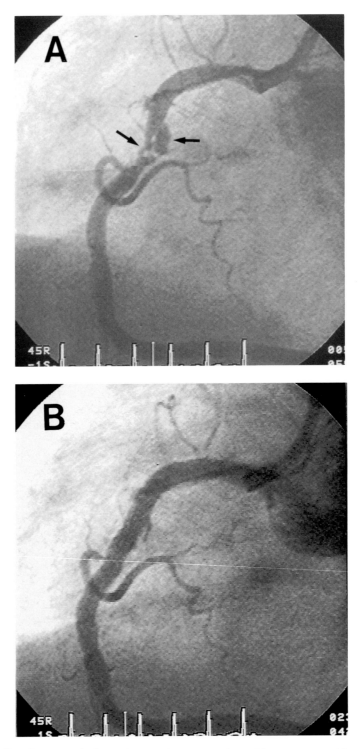

Figure 9.2. A ruptured plaque in a patient presenting with severe unstable angina. (A) Note the severe stenosis in the true lumen (left arrow) and a collection of contrast adjacent to the stenosis (right arrow) connecting to the true lumen. This appearance is classic for plaque rupture. (B) An intracoronary stent was placed at the lesion site, opening the lumen and sealing the ruptured plaque.

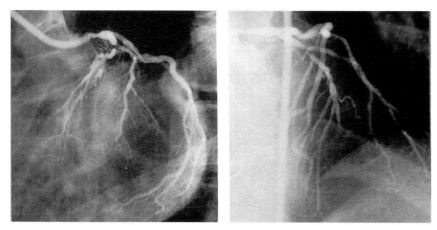

Figure 9.3. Coronary arteriogram of a 52-yr-old male with unstable angina. He presented with frequent episodes of resting chest pain associated with diffuse ST segment depression. The left coronary artery in the left anterior oblique (LAO) (left panel) and right anterior oblique (RAO) (right panel) projections show severe stenoses of the left main, left anterior descending involving a large first diagonal branch, occlusion of the distal left anterior descending, and diffuse disease in the obtuse marginal (as seen in the RAO view).

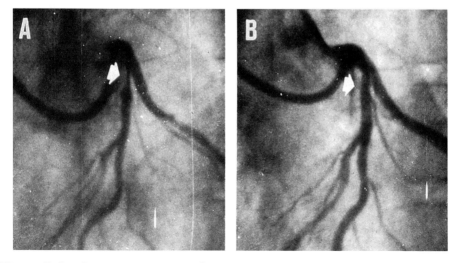

Figure 9.4. Coronary arteriogram of a patient presenting with unstable angina who was found to have coronary artery spasm as its cause. (A) Coronary arteriogram obtained while the patient experienced chest pain shows focal narrowing of the proximal left anterior descending. (B) After nitroglycerin, the spasm is relieved and the artery appears fully patent.

to select one approach or the other, as a combination of both strategies (i.e., planning both a scintigraphic study and a coronary angiogram as a matter of routine) is not an appropriate approach.

Myocardial Infarction

Background

Angiography after myocardial infarction is an area of controversy, in part because of the historical role of coronary angiography as a procedure used in preparation for coronary artery bypass surgery. Since bypass surgery was felt to be contraindicated in patients with recent myocardial infarction, there was initially little need to perform angiography in the weeks after infarction since little would be done with the information. However, demonstrations in the late 1970s of the feasibility of catheterization and bypass surgery during the acute phase of myocardial infarction led to reevaluation of the proscription against these procedures in the postinfarct period.

Specific Settings

Reperfusion Therapy

Angiography in patients with acute myocardial infarction (Figure 9.5) is another area of controversy. It is established that reperfusion therapy, either with direct angioplasty or with thrombolytic therapy, reduces morbidity and mortality associated with the infarction. When a patient is deemed to be a candidate for direct (or "primary") PTCA, it is for obvious reasons necessary to perform angiography prior to performing the PTCA. However, the need for and timing of angiography in patients treated with thrombolytic therapy is less clear. While it might seem intuitive that visualization of the "culprit" lesion will facilitate angioplasty which will in turn prevent reocclusion from occurring in the infarct-related coronary artery, randomized trials performed in the late 1980s showed that such an approach was actually detrimental[29,30] because of an increased rate of femoral access bleeding, which was associated with increased mortality. The situation was compounded by the observation that the degree of lumenal narrowing produced by many lesions decreased significantly over the ensuing week; a significant number of lesions which might have been appropriate targets for PTCA at the time of the initial angiogram regressed to the point where their severity no longer merited intervention.[29] While these observations might suggest that angiography be reserved only for patients who remain unstable and in whom reperfusion is believed to have failed, one study testing a strategy of immediate angiography followed by angioplasty reserved only for totally occluded vessels showed little benefit from this strategy compared with a more conservative strategy.[31]

Another approach which seemed intuitively useful was routine angiography followed by revascularization several days after thrombolytic therapy was given (Figure 9.6). This approach was studied in the second Thrombolysis in Myocardial Infarction study (TIMI II). Patients receiving t-PA within 4 hr of the onset of their infarction were randomized to management with either an "invasive" strategy consisting of routine angiography followed by anatomically directed revascularization 18 to

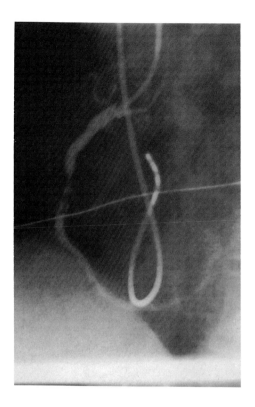

Figure 9.5. Right coronary arteriogram of a patient with an acute myocardial infarction. Note the filling defect in the midcoronary segment indicative of thrombus. Flow beyond the thrombus is sluggish and the distal artery is poorly visualized.

48 hr after the t-PA, or to a "conservative" strategy consisting of exercise radionuclide ventriculography and angiography only for a positive exercise test or recurrent angina or infarction. At 6 wk, 98% of patients in the "invasive" limb and 33% of patients in the "conservative" limb had undergone angiography, but the rates of death or myocardial infarction were identical in both groups (approximately 5% in each limb). The ejection fraction was also identical in both groups.[32] Follow-up at 3 yr shows the same rate of events in both groups.[33] A similar series of strategies was assessed in patients treated with anisoylated plasminogen activator complex (APSAC) in the SWIFT (Should We Intervene Following Thrombolysis?) study, although the angiograms performed in this trial were done at a mean of 5 days after the infarction. Again, there was no difference between the groups in terms of catastrophic events although angina was less common in patients who were randomized to angiography.[34] A third smaller study performed in Israel showed similar findings in patients treated with streptokinase.[35]

Randomized data thus indicate only a small likelihood that routine angiography is useful for the prevention of death or infarction over the few years following thrombolysis. Before these data are accepted as blanket proscriptions against angiography following thrombolysis, two important pieces of data must be reviewed. First, two

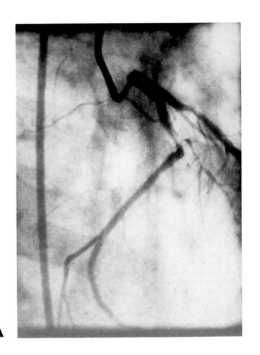

A

Figure 9.6. Left coronary arteriogram of a patient who presented 2 days earlier with an acute inferoposterior myocardial infarction. The patient received t-PA with resolution of symptoms and ST segment abnormalities. (A) RAO projection of the left coronary artery shows a severe residual stenosis in the proximal circumflex as well as a stenotic lesion in the anterior descending. (B) After angioplasty of the culprit lesion, the circumflex is widely patent. The anterior descending lesion was subsequently dilated several weeks later.

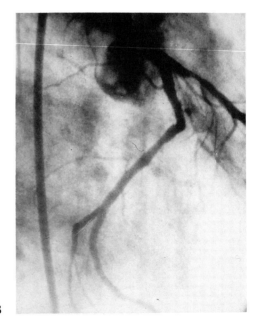

B

174

prospective studies have shown that approximately one-third of vessels in which flow has been restored are occluded 6 months after thrombolysis, regardless of the medical therapy selected.[36,37] It is difficult to explain the relatively low rates of recurrent myocardial infarction reported during this time period if the rate of reocclusion truly is so high. It is possible that if revascularization could be limited to patients in whom substantial amounts of myocardium had been salvaged, recurrent events might be prevented. It is also important to point out that in the studies mentioned above, approximately half of patients would have been eligible for angioplasty based on anatomic information.[32] Two important advances in the area of percutaneous revascularization may lower the likelihood of reocclusion of the infarct vessel. Specifically, the advent of platelet glycoprotein IIb/IIIa inhibitors such as abciximab and the development of intracoronary stents may both prevent reocclusion after angioplasty.[38–40]

A second important consideration is that the aims of angiography in the patient who has undergone thrombolysis need not be limited to prevention of reocclusion of the infarct-related vessel. The identification of patients with multivessel disease who stand to benefit from coronary artery bypass graft surgery requires angiography, and counseling patients regarding risk is also facilitated by knowledge of the angiographic anatomy.

Two other points should be noted. In all of these studies, patients were in generally close proximity to angiographic facilities so that delay was minimal when the need for urgent angiography arose. In substudies of several larger randomized trials, there has been no difference in outcome noted for patients hospitalized at facilities with cardiac catheterization laboratories and those without such equipment.[41,42] It should be remembered that the strategy of "watchful waiting" is predicated on the ability to watch while waiting. When social or geographic circumstances make it difficult to observe patients adequately, a more aggressive approach may be warranted.

Finally, as a result of a concerted effort on the part of paramedical services, emergency room personnel, and treating physicians, the delay in administering thrombolytic therapy after presentation to the emergency room is diminishing.[43] As a result, one would expect that the number of patients with substantial myocardial salvage would increase. Since a small number of patients do show electrocardiographic evidence of rapid and complete reperfusion (i.e., complete return of ST segments to their baseline level), it is unclear whether a more aggressive strategy might be economically more efficient since the likelihood of detecting ischemia might be higher if the extent of myocardial necrosis is reduced.

Patients Without Reperfusion

Because of the interest focused on reperfusion during the last decade, little attention has been paid to patients in whom reperfusion therapy is not given. Current data would indicate that there are substantial numbers of such patients. There have been no large randomized trials to determine whether angiography is indicated in these patients. Again, a combination of symptomatic assessment and noninvasive risk assessment based on nuclear scintigraphic data may help determine a management strategy for such patients. It is clear that patients with ischemic deficits exceeding 15% to 20% of the myocardium are at increased risk for death or reinfarction over the ensuing years.[44] Angiography is thus likely to help identify the vessel responsible for the ischemia and to help plan a revascularization strategy.

Patients With Mechanical Complications

Acute ventricular septal defect and mitral regurgitation complicate approximately 2% of acute myocardial infarctions. Surgical correction of these problems is often essential to survival. In patients with ventricular septal defect, urgent surgery is usually advised while in those with mitral regurgitation, the usual recommendation is to delay surgery if the hemodynamic situation permits. In the latter circumstance, preoperative angiography is mandatory, while emergency angiography in the former is often a luxury. Successful surgery depends on prompt repair of the defect. In this circumstance, angiography should be performed if there is a delay in preparing the operating room or if the patient is hemodynamically stable. Alternatively, it should be realized that abrupt hemodynamic collapse is common in this situation and that angiography may delay achievement of the primary goal which is to support the circulation while the defect is repaired.

Angioplasty Follow-up

When coronary angioplasty was initially performed, most patients underwent angiographic follow-up approximately 6 months after the procedure to determine whether restenosis (Figure 9.7) of the dilated lesion had occurred. Since that time,

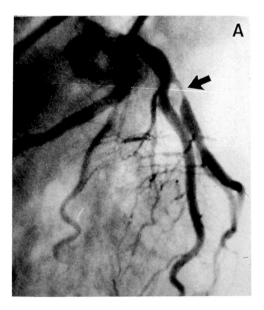

Figure 9.7.   Restenosis, the Achilles heel of angioplasty, is demonstrated in this sequence. (A) A high-grade stenosis of the proximal anterior descending is noted (arrow).

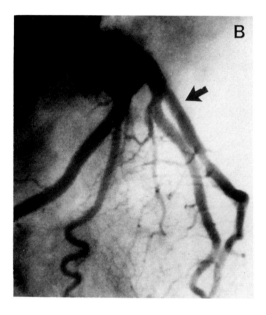

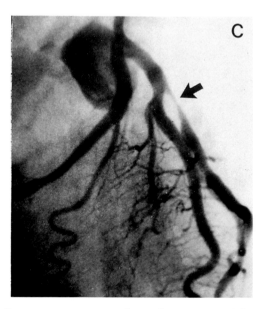

Figure 9.7. (B) Following coronary angioplasty, the artery is widely patent. (C) Symptoms recurred 4 months later. Coronary angiography disclosed restenosis at the prior PTCA site.

however, nuclear scintigraphic techniques have supplanted follow-up angiography in all but the highest risk cases. These cases include patients whose risk for restenosis is above average and who have large amounts of myocardium subserved by the dilated segment. For example, patients who have undergone angioplasty of the proximal portion of the left anterior descending coronary artery and who have complete obstruction in the proximal portion of one of the other major coronary trunks should have follow-up angiography approximately 4 months after the index angioplasty. This time is selected because restenosis is rarely evident before the first month after angioplasty and its incidence reaches a plateau after the fourth month.[45] Another example is the patient who has undergone angioplasty of a saphenous vein graft which supplies the distribution of more than one native coronary artery.

The advent of intracoronary stents has altered the restenosis picture, and arguably has created an entirely new disease process. Two randomized clinical trials have suggested that elective implantation of an intracoronary stent reduces the rate of restenosis,[39,40] and observations suggest that the rate of restenosis can be reduced even further.[46] This lower rate of restenosis might obviate the need to perform repeat angiograms on patients who have undergone angioplasty involving large areas of myocardium. Unfortunately, it has also become clear that the low restenosis rates reported are limited to patients in whom the angioplasty has been performed on relatively discrete lesions. Patients in whom longer lesions have been dilated, or who have extensive dissection requiring repair, often have multiple intracoronary stents implanted (Figure 9.8). The risk of restenosis rises dramatically as the number of implanted stents increases and probably does so as the length of the stented segment increases. Since dilation within a stented segment is performed fairly easily as long as the restenotic lesion is relatively discrete, and while it is much

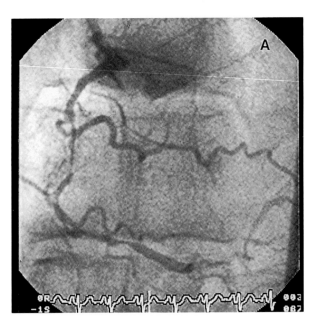

Figure 9.8. Multiple Gianturco-Roubin stents were implanted in this patient with extensive disease in the right coronary artery. A: The coronary artery is severely stenosed almost throughout its course with a seemingly small distal artery distribution.

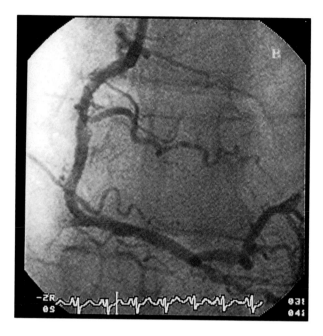

Figure 9.8. B: After stenting, the right coronary artery is widely patent with a large vascular distribution.

more difficult if the lesion progresses to complete occlusion, patients in whom long arterial segments have been stented should undergo routine follow-up arteriography after 3 to 4 months.

Peripheral Vascular Disease

Mortality in patients with peripheral vascular disease most commonly occurs as a result of acute myocardial infarction rather than the peripheral vascular disease itself. As a result, patients scheduled to undergo peripheral vascular surgery often undergo coronary arteriography in preparation. There are, however, few data to support this approach. Several studies have demonstrated that pharmacologic stress combined with nuclear scintigraphy is able to separate patients at high risk of suffering perioperative myocardial infarction from those whose risk is low. On the other hand, patients in whom peripheral vascular surgery of the thoracic aorta is planned probably do stand to benefit from preoperative coronary angiography since this procedure often involves hypothermic circulatory arrest with reimplantation of the coronary ostia.

Noncoronary Cardiac Surgery

Young patients with valvular heart disease are able to undergo open valvular repair without the necessity for coronary angiography. In fact, no catheterization may be needed at all in patients who have simple single valvular lesions (or atrial septal defects) and who have clear echocardiographic findings. However, this is not true of patients with complex congenital heart disease, particularly those with tetralogy of Fallot, since this anomaly is associated with anomalies of the coronary arteries which are subject to the risk of transsection at the time of surgery. Older patients undergoing valvular surgery should have preoperative coronary angiography. Patients with a history of cigarette smoking should undergo arteriography once past the age of 40, and nonsmokers should undergo angiography after the age of 50. Most clinicians would substitute a stress test (either exercise or pharmacologic) for angiography in these patients. Obviously, an angiogram is indicated in patients in whom these noninvasive tests suggest ischemia or in whom angina is present. A strong argument can be mounted to perform coronary angiography in all patients with calcific aortic stenosis. In most studies, approximately half of patients with degenerative aortic stenosis have significant narrowings of the coronary arteries. The pathology of this disease generally involves the aortic root and can extend to the coronary ostia. Such findings are of paramount importance to the cardiac surgeon because of their implications for myocardial preservation during surgery as well as the likelihood that they are ischemia-producing.

Congestive Heart Failure and Heart Transplantation

Despite reductions in the incidence and mortality of acute myocardial infarction in the United States, congestive heart failure continues to grow as a clinical problem. Coronary arteriography is often helpful in establishing an etiology and simplifying a management plan. The likelihood that congestive heart failure is a consequence of coronary artery disease increases with increasing patient age. Consequently, arteriography may be useful in patients with heart failure and multiple risk factors for coronary artery disease, in patients with left ventricular failure who are more than 40 yr old, in patients with electrocardiographic evidence of prior infarction, or in those with angina or provocable ischemia.

Although establishment of the etiologic diagnosis is not likely to be helpful in managing the symptoms of heart failure, it is established that patients with severe multivessel coronary artery disease have prolonged survival after coronary artery bypass, and a variety of adjunctive techniques, including dobutamine echocardiography and combined nuclear perfusion imaging and metabolic studies, have been shown to predict recovery of myocardial function after bypass surgery and are likely to prove helpful for selecting patients for this procedure.

Patients who have undergone heart transplantation pose another difficult situation. Progression of disease in both the epicardial coronary arteries and more distal vasculature occurs in approximately 35% of patients who survive the initial stages of transplantation and is the most common cause of death after the first year following transplantation.[47] Since the heart is surgically denervated at the time of transplantation, organ recipients are generally unable to experience angina. The sensitivity of noninvasive testing in this situation is a matter of controversy. In our own experience, its utility has been limited.[48] Consequently, yearly surveillance angiography is performed in nearly all transplant recipients. Although there is no accepted treatment for the distal coronary arterial narrowings that these patients develop (other than retransplantation), approximately 5% to 10% of patients also develop discrete epicardial narrowings which are amenable to percutaneous revascularization procedures.[49]

SPECIAL CONSIDERATIONS

Resource Utilization and Societal Considerations

Credible data on the frequency with which coronary arteriography is performed today are lacking, however, growth in the number of hospitals with catheterization facilities and the development of mobile coronary catheterization labs would suggest that coronary arteriography has increased dramatically in popularity. At the current time, the best estimate is that approximately 1,000,000 patients per year are believed to undergo coronary arteriography in the United States. In addition to the maturation of coronary artery bypass surgery, several other factors have played important roles in its growth. These include the continuing growth of coronary angioplasty and stent placement, the wider application of more techniques to detect coronary artery disease, such as nuclear scintigraphy and stress echocardiography, the recognition that myocardial "stunning" or postischemic ventricular dysfunction may be reversible by revascularization after myocardial infarction, as well as by the growth in cardiac transplantation and the need for surveillance angiography in patients with denervated hearts. In addition, it is recognized that in other patients ischemia may occur in the absence of symptoms and is associated with a poor prognosis. Another important factor in the growth of coronary angiography has been its conversion from an inpatient procedure requiring 1 to 2 days of hospitalization to an outpatient procedure requiring a hospital or outpatient catheterization center stay as brief as 3 to 4 hr.

Within North America and Europe, considerable variations exist in the use of coronary arteriography. For example, patients hospitalized in a facility where coronary angiography is available are approximately three times more likely to undergo catheterization than patients who were hospitalized at a hospital without a catheterization laboratory.[50] In a review of the 1990 Medicare database, 30% of patients in New York State underwent a cardiac catheterization within 90 days of a myocardial infarction compared with 45% of patients in Texas.[51] In contrast, a study of patients enrolled in the Global Utilization of Streptokinase and Tissue Plasminogen Activator for Occluded Coronary Arteries (GUSTO) trial of treatments for myocardial infarction examined eight regions in the United States. The frequency with which coronary angiography was performed prior to hospital discharge after infarction was higher than predicted using a multivariate model derived from patient characteristics but was constant throughout the country. On the other hand, the availability of angiographic facilities was a more powerful predictor of the likelihood of having angiography. However, in all the models tested, angiography was less likely to be performed on patients in New England than in other parts of the country.[52]

Until recently, the international variation in the use of coronary angiography was even greater than that in the United States. In the GUSTO study, cardiac catheterization facilities were available at 41% of hospitals in Canada compared with 77% in the United States.[53] Consequently, 25% of patients enrolled in Canada had angiography prior to hospital discharge compared with 72% in the United States.[54,55] In Europe, usage of angiography was also lower than in the United States. However, it appears that coronary angiography is increasing in popularity in most countries. In the Multinational Monitoring of Trends and Determinants in Cardiovascular Disease (MONICA) study of myocardial infarction, for example, 68.2% of patients with acute myocardial infarction in southeastern France underwent angiography in 1986 compared with 87.3% in 1990.[56] This technology diffusion is probably the result of the same forces that have increased the popularity of angiography in the United States—the ease with which the procedure can be performed, the number of angiographers completing training programs, the availability of mobile catheterization laboratories, the extension of PTCA to patients for whom revascularization had not previously been an option, as well as remuneration systems that provide incentive to refer patients for angiography.

FUTURE CONSIDERATIONS

Cineless Image Processing

Advances in digital image technology have led to the ability to record images in digital format and storage on magnetic media rather than in the analog form required to store images on photographic media. This "cineless" digital imaging has gained increasing popularity for several reasons. First, processing of images using digital techniques consists of electronic transfer of files rather than "wet" darkroom technology, and thus is potentially less expensive and less time-consuming. Second, archiving of angiographic information takes considerably less physical storage space when magnetic media are used. Third, "postprocessing", i.e., modification of images and reproduction of still frames, is accomplished much more easily when magnetic media are used. Finally, transfer of images can be performed electronically over Ethernet connections, or integrated systems digital network (ISDN) lines rather than mailing of 35-mm films. The bandwidth of standard telephone lines will not allow sufficiently rapid data transfer. It is thus conceivable that a cardiologist will be able to view cineangiograms for a patient on a monitor located in his office, while the actual files are stored at remote location.

SUMMARY AND CONCLUSIONS

Coronary angiography has become one of the major diagnostic tools in the medical armamentarium. The malicious nature of coronary artery disease has prompted the advancement of coronary angiography to the point where it is a highly reliable diagnostic tool and can be performed with extremely low morbidity and mortality. Currently, it provides the most definitive diagnosis of clinically significant coronary artery disease. Its utility is established in virtually all aspects of the coronary artery disease spectrum although the specific indications and urgency to perform coronary angiography vary depending upon the clinical presentation.

While this chapter focused on a discussion of the specific indications and uses of coronary angiography, an important premise in the management of patients suspected or known to have coronary artery disease is that coronary angiography should be performed in any patient and at any time there is, in the clinical judgment of the responsible physician, a "need to know" the coronary anatomy.

REFERENCES

1. Hurst JAW: *Notes from a Chairman*. Chicago, Year Book Medical Publishers, 1987.
2. Gregg D: The George E. Brown memorial lecture: physiology of the coronary circulation. *Circulation* 28:1128–1137, 1963.
3. Gould K, Lipscomb K, Hamilton G: Physiologic basis for assessing critical coronary stenosis. *Am J Cardiol* 1974;33:87–94.
4. Proudfit W, Shirey E, Sones FJ: Selective cine coronary arteriography: correlation with clinical findings in 1000 patients. *Circulation* 1966;33:901.
5. Proudfit W, Shirey E, Sheldon W, et al: Certain clinical characteristics correlated with extent of obstructive lesions demonstrated by selective cine-coronary arteriography. *Circulation* 1968;38:947.
6. Koza MJ, Shankey TC, Walenga JM, et al: Flow cytometric evaluation of platelet activation by ionic or nonionic contrast media and modulation by heparin and recombinant hirudin. *Invest Radiol* 1995;30:90–97.
7. Granger CB, Gabriel DA, Reece NS, et al: Fibrin modification by ionic and nonionic contrast media during cardiac catheterization. *Am J Cardiol* 1992;69:821–823.
8. Sheu SH, Hang MH, Piao ZE, et al: Effects of contrast media on coronary hemodynamics and myocardial metabolism. *Invest. Radiol.* 1995 30(1):28–32.
9. Manske CL, Sprafka JMU, Strony JT, et al: Contrast nephropathy in azotemic diabetic patients undergoing coronary angiography. *Am J Med.* 1990;89:615–620.
10. Solomon R, Werner C, Mann D, et al: Effects of saline, mannitol, and furosemide to prevent acute decreases in renal function induced by radiocontrast agents. *N Engl J Med* 1994;331:1416–1420.
11. Roberts WC, Jones AA: Quantitation of coronary arterial narrowing at necropsy in sudden coronary death: analysis of 31 patients and comparison with 25 control subjects. *Am J Cardiol* 1979;44:39–45.
12. Arnett EN, Isner JM, Redwood DR, et al: Coronary artery narrowing in coronary heart disease: comparison of cineangiographic and necropsy findings. *Ann. Intern. Med.* 1979;91:350–356.
13. Nishimura RA, Edwards WD, Warnes CA, et al: Intravascular ultrasound imaging: in vitro validation and pathologic correlation. *J Am Coll Cardiol* 1990;16:145–154.
14. Potkin BN, Bartorelli AL, Gessert JM, et al: Coronary artery imaging with intravascular high-frequency ultrasound. *Circulation* 1990;81:1575–1585.
15. Vlodaver Z, Frech R, Van Tassel RA, et al: Correlation of the antemortem coronary arteriogram and the postmortem specimen. *Circulation* 1973;47:162–169.
16. Zir LM, Miller SW, Dinsmore RE, et al: Interobserver variability in coronary angiography. *Circulation* 53:627–632, 1976.

17. Reiber J, Kooijman C, Slager C, et al: Coronary artery dimensions from cineangiograms—methodology and validation of a computer assisted analysis procedure. *IIEE Trans. Med. Imaging* 1984;MI-3:131–141.

18. Kemp H, Kronmal R, Viletstra D, Frye R, and participants in the coronary artery surgery study: Seven year survival of patients with normal or near normal coronary arteriograms: a CASS Registry Study. *J Am Coll Cardiol* 1986;7:479–483.

19. McKenna W, Deanfield J, Faruqui A, et al: Prognosis in hypertrophic cardiomyopathy: role of age and clinical, electrocardiographic and hemodynamic features. *Am J Cardiol* 1981;47:532–538.

20. CASS Investigators: Myocardial infarction and mortality in the Coronary Artery Surgery Study (CASS) randomized trial. *N Engl J Med* 1984;310:750–758.

21. Parisi AF, Folland ED, Hartigan P: A comparison of angioplasty with medical therapy in the treatment of single-vessel coronary artery disease. Veterans Affairs ACME Investigators. *N Engl J Med* 1992;326:10–16.

22. Rogers WJ, Bourassa MG, Andrews TC, et al: Asymptomatic Cardiac Ischemia Pilot (ACIP) study: outcome at 1 year for patients with asymptomatic cardiac ischemia randomized to medical therapy or revascularization. The ACIP Investigators. *J Am Coll Cardiol* 1995;26:594–605.

23. Mark DB, Hlatky MA, Califf RM, et al: Cost effectiveness of thrombolytic therapy with tissue plasminogen activator as compared with streptokinase for acute myocardial infarction. *N Engl J Med* 1995;332:1418–1424.

24. Braunwald E: Unstable angina. A classification. *Circulation* 1989;80:410–414.

25. van Miltenburg-van Zijl AJ, Simoons ML, Veerhoek RJ, et al: Incidence and follow-up of Braunwald subgroups in unstable angina pectoris. *J Am Coll Cardiol* 1995;25:1286–1292.

26. The TIMI IIIB Investigators: Effects of tissue plasminogen activator and a comparison of early invasive and conservative strategies in unstable angina and non-Q-wave myocardial infarction: results of the TIMI IIIB trial. *Circulation* 1994;89:1545–1556.

27. Anderson HV, Cannon CP, Stone PH, et al: One-year results of the Thrombolysis in Myocardial Infarction (TIMI) IIIB clinical trial. A randomized comparison of tissue-type plasminogen activator versus placebo and early invasive versus early conservative strategies in unstable angina and non-Q wave myocardial infarction. *J Am Coll Cardiol* 1995;26:1643–1650.

28. TIMI IIIA Investigators: Early effects of tissue-type plasminogen activator added to conventional therapy on the culprit coronary lesion in patients presenting with ischemic cardiac pain at rest: results of the Thrombolysis in Myocardial Ischemia (TIMI IIIA) trial. *Circulation* 1993;87:38–52.

29. Rogers W, Baim D, Gore J: Comparison of immediate invasive, delayed invasive, and conservative strategies after tissue-type plasminogen activator: results of the Thrombolysis in Myocardial Infarction (TIMI) phase II-A trial. *Circulation* 81:1457–1476, 1990.

30. Topol E, Califf R, George B: A randomized trial of immediate versus delayed elective angioplasty after intravenous tissue plasminogen activator in acute myocardial infarction. *N Engl J Med* 1987;317:581–588.

31. Califf RM, Topol EJ, Stack RS, et al: Evaluation of combination thrombolytic therapy and timing of cardiac catheterization in myocardial infarction. Results of the Thrombolysis and Angioplasty in Myocardial Infarction–phase 5 trial. *Circulation* 1992;83:1543–1556.

32. The TIMI Study Group: Comparison of invasive and conservative strategies after treatment with intravenous tissue plasminogen activator in acute myocardial infarction. Rests

of the Thrombolysis in Myocardial Infarction (TIMI) phase II trial. *N Engl J Med* 1989;320:618–627.

33. Terrin ML, Williams DO, Kleiman NS, et al: Two- and three-year results of the Thrombolysis in Myocardial Infarction (TIMI) phase II clinical trial. *J Am Coll Cardiol* 1993;22:1763–1772.

34. SWIFT (Should We Intervene Following Thrombolysis?) Trial Study Group: SWIFT trial of delayed elective intervention v conservative treatment after thrombolysis with anistreptase in acute myocardial infarction. *BMJ* 1991;302:555–560.

35. Barbash GI, Roth A, Hod H, et al: Randomized controlled trial of late in-hospital angiography and angioplasty versus conservative management after treatment with recombinant tissue-type plasminogen activator in acute myocardial infarction. *Am J Cardiol* 1990;66:538–545.

36. White HD, French JK, Hamer AW, et al: Frequent reocclusion of patent infarct-related arteries between 4 weeks and 1 year: effects of antiplatelet therapy. *J Am Coll Cardiol* 1995;25:218–223.

37. Meijer A, Verheugt FW, Werter CJ, et al: Aspirin versus coumadine in the prevention of reocclusion and recurrent ischemia after successful thrombolysis: a prospective placebo-controlled angiographic study. Results of the APRICOT study. *Circulation* 1993;87:1524–1530.

38. The EPIC Investigators: Use of a monoclonal antibody directed against the platelet glycoprotein IIb/IIIa receptor in high-risk coronary angioplasty. *N Engl J Med* 1994;330:956–961.

39. Serruys PW, de Jaegre P, Kiemeneij F, et al: A comparison of balloon-expandable stent implantation with balloon angioplasty in patients with coronary artery disease. *N Engl J Med* 1994;331:489–495.

40. Fischman DL, Leon MB, Baim DS, et al: A randomized comparison of coronary-stent placement and balloon angioplasty in the treatment of coronary artery disease. *N Engl J Med* 1994;331:496–501.

41. White HD, Modan M, Diaz R, Hampton JR, et al: Outcome of thrombolytic therapy in relation to hospital size and invasive cardiac services. The Investigators of the International Tissue Plasminogen Activator/Streptokinase Mortality Trial. *Arch. Intern. Med.* 154: 2237–2242, 1994.

42. Feit F, Mueller HS, Ross Rald E, et al: Thrombolysis in Myocardial Infarction (TIMI) phase II trial: outcome comparison of a "conservative strategy" in community versus tertiary hospitals. The TIMI Research Group. *J Am Coll Cardiol* 1990 16(7):1529–1534.

43. Rogers WJ, Bowby LJ, Chandra NC, et al: Treatment of myocardial infarction in the United States (1990 to 1993). Observations from the National Registry of Myocardial infarction. *Circulation* 1990;90:2103–2114.

44. Mahmarian JJ, Mahmarian AC, Marks GF, et al: Role of adenosine thallium-201 tomography for defining long-term risk in patients after acute myocardial infarction. *J Am Coll Cardiol* 1995;25:1333–1340.

45. Nobuyoshi M, Kimura T, Nosaka H, et al: Restenosis after successful percutaneous transluminal coronary angioplasty: serial angiographic follow-up of 229 patients. *J Am Coll Cardiol* 1988;12:616–623.

46. Serruys PW, Emanuelsson H, Lunn AC, et al: Heparin-coated Palmaz-Schatz stents in human coronary arteries. Early outcome of the Benestent-II Pilot Study. *Circulation* 1996;93:412–422.

47. Young JB, Smart FM, Lowry RL, et al: Coronary angiography after heart transplanta-

tion: should preoperative study be the "gold standard"? *J Heart Lung Transplant* 1992; 11(Pt 2):S65–68.

48. Smart FW, Ballantyne CM, Cocanougher B, et al: Insensitivity of non-invasive tests to detect coronary artery vasculopathy after heart transplant. *Am J Cardiol* 1991;67: 243–247(Abstract).

49. Verani MS, Taillefer R, Mahmarian JJ, et al: for the IPPA Study Group: I-23 Iodophenylpentadecanoic acid (IPPA) metabolic imaging predicts improvement of global left ventricular function after coronary revascularization. *J Am Coll Cardiol* 1996;27(suppl): 300A.

50. Halle AA 3rd, Diciascio G, Massin EK, et al: Coronary angioplasty, atherectomy and bypass surgery in cardiac transplant recipients. *J Am Coll Cardiol* 1995;26:120–128.

51. Every NR, Larson EB, Litwin PE, et al: The association between on-site cardiac catheterization facilities and the use of coronary angiography after acute myocardial infarction. Myocardial Infarction Triage and Intervention Project investigators. *N Engl J Med* 329:546–551, 1993.

52. Guadagnoli E, Hauptman PJ, Ayanian JZ et al: Variation in the use of cardiac procedures after acute myocardial infarction. *N Engl J Med* 1995;333:573–578.

53. Pilote L, Califf RM, Sapp S, et al: Regional variation across the United States in the management of acute myocardial infarction. GUSTO-1 Investigators. Global Utilization of Streptokinase and Tissue Plasminogen Activator for Occluded Coronary Arteries. *N Engl J Med* 1995;333:565–572.

54. Pilote L, Granger C, Armstrong P, et al: Differences in the treatment of myocardial infarction between the United States and Canada. A survey of physicians in the GUSTO trial. *Med Care* 1996;33:598–610.

55. Mark DB, Naylor CD, Hlatky MA, et al: Use of medical resources and quality of life after acute myocardial infarction in Canada and the United States. *N Engl J Med* 1994; 331:1130–1135.

56. Ferrieres J, Cambou J-P, Ruidavets J-B, Pous J: "Trends in acute myocardial infarction prognosis and treatment in southwestern France between 1985 and 1990 (The MONICA project-Toulouse). *Am J Cardiol* 75:1202–1205, 1995.

— 10 —

Noncardiac Angiography

Albert E. Raizner, M.D.

Traditionally, a division of responsibility has existed between the invasive cardiologist and the invasive radiologist. The invasive cardiologist, whose attention is clearly directed to the evaluation of cardiac disorders, has generally had a tangential exposure to the evaluation of noncardiac disease. The invasive radiologist, on the other hand, has focused his or her attention to the evaluation of noncardiac disorders, including the angiographic evaluation of pulmonary, aortic, and peripheral vascular diseases.

This "division of labor," however, is artefactual when clinical perspectives are considered. For example, patients with coronary atherosclerotic disease often have atherosclerotic disease of peripheral vessels, such as the carotid arteries, aorta, and arteries of the iliofemoral system. Additionally, patients presenting with manifestations of noncardiac vascular disease states, such as aortic aneurysm, carotid and peripheral vascular disease, will often require assessment of their coronary circulation, particularly if surgical intervention is anticipated.

Consequently, the cardiologist's role has been expanded to include noncardiac vascular disease, often, but not exclusively, in conjunction with the evaluation of the heart. This chapter will discuss the most common noncardiac angiography procedures which are performed by the cardiologist. Additionally, it behooves the internists and primary care physicians to have an understanding of the indications for requesting noncardiac angiography in conjunction with invasive cardiac evaluation.

187

DESCRIPTION OF TECHNIQUE

This chapter will focus solely on catheter-based techniques. The reader is directed to the chapters on Echocardiography (Chapter 1), Magnetic Resonance Imaging (Chapter 4), and Transesophageal Echocardiography (Chapter 6) in which some aspects of nonangiographic imaging of noncardiac vascular structures are discussed.

Included in the discussion will be those techniques which are most commonly utilized in conjunction with invasive cardiac angiography: (1) aortography, including the study of the ascending aorta, aortic arch, descending thoracic aorta, and abdominal aorta; (2) carotid angiography; (3) subclavian angiography; (4) renal angiography; and (5) peripheral angiography involving the iliac and femoral arteries.

DEVELOPMENTAL PERSPECTIVES

In 1895, Wilhelm Konrad Roentgen, while working with a cathode ray tube (similar to a conventional television tube) noted that it lit up a fluorescent screen which was several feet away. Since cathode rays were known to travel only a short distance, the activation of the fluorescent screen had to have been done by another type of ray beam. Roentgen designated it the "x-ray"; the "x" referring to the fact that the nature of this beam was unknown. Thus, the world of x-ray technology was discovered and, too, its vast potential for diagnosing medical diseases.

Shortly thereafter, the first arteriogram was performed in 1896 by Hascheck and Lindenthal. They injected barium into a cadaver artery while obtaining an x-ray image of the structure.

The first recorded catheter insertion in a human was performed by Werner Forssmann in 1929.[1] However, it was not until Seldinger[2] developed a method for the percutaneous entry of a catheter into a peripheral artery in 1953 that the technique of arteriography as a clinically useful method for the diagnosis of arterial diseases was initiated. Since that time, arteriography has developed to the point where the modern invasive cardiologist or radiologist can visualize virtually any artery in the human body.

TECHNICAL CONSIDERATIONS

Contrast angiography of the aorta and peripheral vessels may employ a variety of catheter techniques, contrast agents, and radiographic techniques.

To access the arterial circulation, percutaneous puncture of the femoral artery is the most common approach utilized. However, access of the brachial artery via percutaneous puncture or cutdown is still used in many laboratories and may be the only means of access in some clinical circumstances such as occlusion of the distal aorta or of both iliac arteries. Most commonly, 5-Fr or 6-Fr catheters are used, the latter providing better contrast flow rates particularly when hand injections are utilized.

Ionic contrast agents are utilized in most laboratories for use in the aorta or peripheral circulation. Their lower cost relative to nonionic contrast agents favors their use in most angiographic laboratories.[3] The nonionic contrast agents, however, are better tolerated and are associated with fewer side effects.[4] The addition of lidocaine to either contrast agent lessens the discomfort associated with these agents.

Radiographic techniques vary widely and each has advantages and disadvantages. Large serial cut films provide a large field of view, up to $14'' \times 14''$, and provide very high resolution. Cineangiography is most commonly used when peripheral angiography is combined with cardiac catheterization and coronary angiography in a cardiac catheterization laboratory. It offers the advantage of viewing structures in motion and allowing the area of visualization to be extended by panning along the flow of contrast media. Digital acquisition has become increasingly popular and may ultimately replace either of the aforementioned techniques. It offers the advantages of image processing, use of less contrast media, and ease of subtraction techniques for image enhancement. Digital acquisition is ideal for use in interventional procedures because of its ability to serve as a road map and for the online comparison of pre and post images.

INDICATIONS AND USES

Virtually every major artery in the human body can be selectively or subselectively catheterized and arteriograms obtained. In this section, we will review the major arterial structures and arterial systems which, in clinical practice, most commonly undergo arteriographic study (Tables 10.1 and 10.2).

Ascending Aortography

Aortic Valve Disease

Ascending aortography is invaluable in the assessment of aortic valve disease. Patients with aortic stenosis commonly exhibit dilatation of the ascending aorta.[5] Occasionally, this dilatation reaches aneurysmal proportions, particularly if combined aortic stenosis and regurgitation are present. Ascending aortography allows quantitation of the degree of dilatation and the extent of involvement of the ascending aorta.

Supravalvular aortic stenosis requires both hemodynamic and angiographic assessment to fully define its severity and the feasibility of surgical correction. The angiographic finding of constriction of the aorta beginning above the aortic valve, combined with a pressure gradient as the catheter is withdrawn through the ascending aorta, establishes the diagnosis.[6]

Localization of the aortic valve ostium is occasionally needed to facilitate passage of the catheter into the left ventricle to ascertain the severity of aortic valve stenosis. This technique is sometimes necessary in patients undergoing balloon aortic valvuloplasty.

TABLE 10.1.   Indications and Uses of Aortography

  I. Ascending aortography
      1. Aortic regurgitation
      2. Supravalvular aortic stenosis
      3. Ascending aortic aneurysm
      4. Annuloaortic ectasia
      5. Aneurysms of sinuses of Valsalva
      6. Dissection of the aorta
      7. Coronary bypass grafts
      8. Anomalous origin of coronary arteries
      9. Infective endocarditis
 II. Arch aortography
      1. Dissection of the aorta
      2. Disease of the great vessels
III. Descending aortography
      1. Descending thoracic aortic aneurysms
      2. Coarction of the aorta
      3. Traumatic aneurysms; aortic transection
 IV. Abdominal aortography
      1. Abdominal aortic aneurysms
      2. Dissection of the aorta
      3. Atherosclerotic obstructive disease
          a. Leriche's syndrome
          b. Intestinal ischemic syndromes
      4. Supported coronary angioplasty

TABLE 10.2.   Indications and Uses of Selected Peripheral Arteriography

  I. Renal arteriography
      1. Renal artery stenosis
      2. Abrupt and unexplained renal failure
      3. Renal mass
 II. Iliofemoral arteriography
      1. Intermittent claudication
III. Carotid arteriography
      1. Carotid artery bruits
      2. Transient ischemic attacks (TIAs)
 IV. Subclavian arteriography
      1. Upper extremity claudication
      2. Subclavian steal syndrome
      3. Myocardial ischemia in patient with internal mammary artery bypass

Perhaps the most common use of ascending aortography in conjunction with cardiac catheterization is the semiquantitative assessment of the degree of severity of aortic regurgitation[7] (Figure 10.1). A grading system of 1–4 is utilized, with 1 indicating trivial regurgitation (a small puff which clears with the subsequent left ventricular contraction), grade 2 mild (regurgitant dye which gradually increases the contrast content of the left ventricle but requiring more than two beats to equalize with aortic contrast), grade 3 moderate (same as 2 but contrast equalizes within two heartbeats), and grade 4 severe (full opacification of the left ventricle is achieved during the first diastolic period) regurgitation.[8] This method of assessing aortic regurgitation, however, has limitations and may be misleading in a patient with a markedly enlarged aorta and left ventricle, a patient with poor left ventricular systolic ejection, and when contrast injection or x-ray visualization is suboptimal.

Aortic Aneurysm

Aortic aneurysms may be caused by atherosclerosis,[9] hereditary defects such as Marfan's syndrome, or may be caused by inflammation or infection. Calcification of the aortic wall in conjunction with an aneurysm is most commonly observed in atherosclerotic and luetic aneurysms.

Patients with Marfan's syndrome,[10] or those who have a forme fruste of Marfan's, may present with dilatation of the ascending aorta on a chest x-ray or fortu-

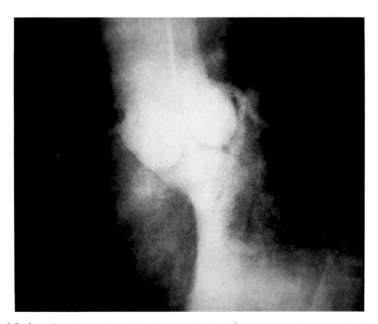

Figure 10.1. Aortic root injection in a patient with severe aortic regurgitation. There is full opacification of the left ventricle within two full cardiac cycles, consistent with severe (3/4) regurgitation.

itously detected during echocardiography. When the ascending aorta alone is involved, the term *idiopathic annuloaortic ectasia* may be applied. In patients with Marfan's or with annuloaortic ectasia, the dilatation usually begins at the aortic valve annulus and involves all three sinuses of Valsalva. Aortic valve function is frequently affected with various degrees of aortic regurgitation detectable.

Aortic Dissection

Patients with aortic dissection often present with a characteristic clinical picture of very severe and unrelenting chest, back, or abdominal pain in conjunction with marked hypertension. Others, however, present with more subtle findings. The DeBakey classification of aortic dissections include Type I (involvement of the ascending, arch and descending thoracic aorta often extending into the abdominal aorta) (Figure 10.2), Type II (involvement of ascending aorta alone), and Type III (dissection beginning in the descending thoracic aorta).[11] Complete angiographic assessment of the entire aorta (total aortography) is often needed in patients with aortic dissection to fully define the entry point and extent of dissection, as well as involvement of important branch vessels. These points of information are crucial in

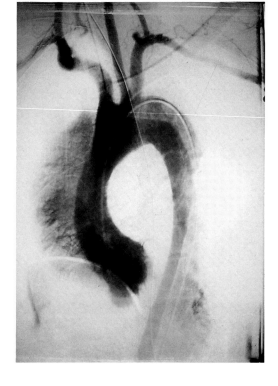

Figure 10.2. Dissection of the aorta. The dissection begins in the ascending aorta and extends to the aortic arch and descending thoracic aorta. This patient subsequently underwent successful two-stage repair of the aortic dissection. (Courtesy of Dr. Joseph Coselli, Houston, Texas.)

planning a surgical strategy. Acute dissection involving the ascending aorta is particularly precarious because of the proximity to the pericardial reflexion, resulting in acute tamponade and often death, involvement of the coronary arteries resulting in myocardial infarction, or extension to the great vessels in the arch leading to stroke.

The angiographic demonstration of an intimal flap or a false lumen establishes the diagnosis.[12,13] A steep left anterior oblique (LAO) angulation is the most useful single plane view. Biplane visualization (LAO/RAO or anteroposterior [AP]/lateral) decreases the likelihood of missing the correct diagnosis.

Bypass Graft Visualization

A large population of patients who have undergone prior coronary bypass surgery exists. The recurrence of ischemic problems in such patients often demands angiographic assessment of the patency of the bypass grafts. While selective visualization of patent grafts is necessary to fully define the presence and extent of disease in the graft, occasionally, the ostium of the graft is difficult to find by blind catheter technique. Ascending aortography is extremely helpful in assessing the location as well as the patency of the grafts. Often, LAO and RAO views are necessary.

Anomalous Coronary Arteries

The finding of anomalous coronary arteries is often established fortuitously during the course of selective coronary angiography.[14] The inability to locate the coronary artery in the anticipated location is a clue to the presence of an anomalous origin. Ascending aortography in at least two views may be helpful in defining the origin and course of the anomalous vessel. When the anomalous artery runs between the pulmonary artery and the aorta, constriction of the artery by these structures may produce ischemic manifestations.

Infective Endocarditis

Patients with infective endocarditis of the aortic valve should undergo ascending aortography to define the severity of valve dysfunction (regurgitation) and, perhaps more importantly, to assess the presence of abscesses or abscess tracks leading to other cardiac chambers. The precise definition of these abscesses or tracks is necessary for complete and proper surgical management since leaving an undetected track will usually result in recurrent infection after surgery.[15] In patients with infective aortic endocarditis, experience, skill, and judgment of the angiographer are required for the safe performance of the study.

Arch Aortography

Aortic Dissection

Involvement of the aortic arch in DeBakey Type I dissection can be a particularly devastating clinical problem. Massive stroke and death may ensue if the innominate artery or left common carotid artery is completely occluded by the dissection.[16]

More commonly, partial obstruction by extension of the arch dissection into the great vessels occurs leading to variable degrees of cerebral ischemia. Precise definition of the degree and extent of involvement of the arch vessels is necessary as urgent surgical correction is required when cerebral flow is compromised. Visualization of the great vessels is best seen in a steep LAO view.

Determination of the Location of the Great Vessels

Selective cannulation of any one of the great vessels requires determination of its origin. In most instances, an experienced angiographer can "feel" for the origin. Occasionally, however, an unusual or anomalous origin or common origin of two of the great vessels may make selective cannulation difficult. Arch aortography will help locate and define the anatomic variation in these cases.

Evaluation of Stenosis of the Great Vessels

Stenosis of the origin of one or more of the great vessels is not uncommon. Of the arch vessels, stenosis of the left subclavian is more common than innominate or left common carotid artery stenosis. Selective cannulation of the great vessels may be misleading in the face of ostial stenosis since the catheter tip may extend distal to the stenosis. Contrast injection in these instances may fail to reveal a clinically important problem. Lack of regurgitation of contrast into the arch during catheter injection, or damping of pressure at the catheter tip suggests an ostial stenosis. Arch aortography in a steep LAO projection will allow angiographic visualization of the stenotic lesion.

Descending Aortography

Descending Thoracic Aortic Aneurysms

Atherosclerotic aortic aneurysms are often located in the descending thoracic aorta just distal to the origin of the left subclavian artery (Figure 10.3). Such aneurysms are often suspected from a chest x-ray showing an excess bulge of the left mediastinum. Type I and III aortic dissections also involve the descending thoracic aorta. Visualization of aneurysms of the descending thoracic aorta is best obtained in a steep LAO projection or combined with a biplane RAO view.

Coarctation of the Aorta

The diagnosis of aortic coarctation is usually made or suspected from clinical features,[17] particularly lower pressures in the lower extremities. Complete assessment of a coarctation requires hemodynamic and angiographic assessment. The location and length of the coarct and the nature and extent of collateral vessels may be determined by aortography. In most instances of coarctation, retrograde catheterization via a femoral artery is adequate. Occasionally, this approach does not allow passage of the catheter through the coarct. In these circumstances, left or right brachial artery cannulation is necessary.

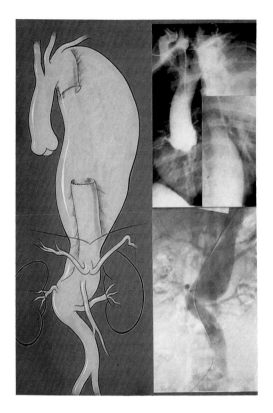

Figure 10.3. Aneurysm involving the descending thoracic aorta and abdominal aorta. (Courtesy of Dr. Joseph Coselli, Houston, Texas.)

Traumatic Aneurysms

Blood or penetrating injuries may damage the aorta. Blunt trauma such as steering wheel injuries to the chest may result in partial or complete transection of the aorta since the aorta is fixed to the chest wall at the aortic isthmus distal to the origin of the left subclavian artery.[18] Aortography is crucial in the assessment of the extent of transection. Surgical intervention is required in all patients.[19]

Abdominal Aortography

Abdominal Aortic Aneurysms

While computed tomography and magnetic resonance imaging have generally supplanted abdominal aortography as the method of choice in assessing the size of abdominal aortic aneurysms, abdominal aortography provides invaluable information regarding the extent of the aneurysm and involvement of major branch vessels, including the renal arteries, superior mesenteric, and the common iliac arteries. Currently, there is a great deal of interest among interventionalists in the potential for the treatment of aortic aneurysms with an intraluminal stent–graft combination. The precise delineation of "healthy" aortic margins proximal and distal to the aneurysm is necessary if this new therapeutic approach is to be successful. Currently, aortography is the only method of obtaining such precise information.

Aortic Dissection

Involvement of the abdominal aorta as well as the thoracic aorta in the dissection process is common. Furthermore, surgical repair of thoracoabdominal aneurysms, in experienced hands, can be undertaken with an acceptably low mortality. Aortography generally provides superior information regarding branch vessel involvement in the dissection process.[20] Surgical repair of the abdominal component of the aortic dissection usually entails the reimplantation of involved branches into the graft.

Atherosclerotic Obstructive Disease

Knowledge of the extent, location, and severity of atherosclerotic involvement of the distal aorta is required in a variety of clinical circumstances. Patients with bilateral hip and buttock claudication (Leriche syndrome) generally have disease involving the distal aorta as well as the proximal segments of the common iliac arteries. A decision to treat by interventional methods or bypass surgery requires arteriographic definition and localization of the intraluminal disease.

Patients who are likely to require an intra-aortic balloon pump as support during a coronary angioplasty or in conjunction with coronary bypass surgery would benefit from preprocedural or preoperative aortoiliac angiography to assess the adequacy and patency of the arteries through which the intra-aortic balloon is to be passed. The same is true if cardiopulmonary support is to be considered in patients undergoing high-risk coronary angioplasty.

In patients undergoing balloon aortic valvuloplasty, aortography of the distal aorta and iliac arteries is routinely performed to ascertain the least tortuous and most patent route for passage of the bulky, high-profile balloon catheters used in this procedure.

Renal Arteriography

Nonselective and selective renal arteriography is occasionally required for the evaluation of hypertension.[21,22] Cardiology practices have varied widely regarding the concomitant use of renal arteriography in hypertensive patients who are undergoing cardiac catheterization. In such patients, renal arteriography is indicated if: (a) the hypertension is moderately severe and is of abrupt or recent onset; (b) there has been a recent and unexplained worsening of hypertension; (c) the patient is young, and, in particular, a younger female patient; (d) a patient with longstanding hypertension has become refractory to first- and second-line antihypertensive medications.

Abdominal aortography alone, particularly when viewed only in an anteroposterior projection, may be misleading due to overlap of the aorta with the generally ostial location of renal atherosclerotic disease. Consequently, selective right and left renal arteriograms are often necessary for accurate evaluation of the severity of renal artery stenosis (Figure 10.4).

Iliofemoral Angiography

The accessibility of the femoral arteries, as well as the arteries below the knee (anterior and posterior tibial, and peroneal), to interventional techniques has made arteriography of the iliofemoral system a commonly used technique (Figure 10.5). The coexistence of symptomatic peripheral vascular disease and coronary artery disease provides common justification for the performance of peripheral arteriography in patients undergoing coronary angiography. Traditional single-plane cardiac catheterization laboratories are unable to assess the coronary circulation as well as the circulation in the lower legs unless the patient is turned upside down to study the peripheral circulation after the coronary angiograms are obtained. The recent development of ceiling-mounted systems has obviated this shortcoming and allowed "head-to-toe" arteriographic study without awkward positioning of the patient.

Carotid Arteriography

Just as the coexistence of peripheral vascular disease involving the lower extremities with coronary artery disease dictates the performance of peripheral angiography in patients undergoing cardiac catheterization, so, too, the common coexistence of carotid artery disease mandates arteriographic study of the extracranial carotid arteries during the course of cardiac catheterization in certain patients. Carotid arteriography[23] should be performed in patients with transient ischemic attacks (TIAs) attributable to the internal carotid arterial circulation, patients with amaurosis fugax, and patients with ultrasound evidence of significant carotid artery stenosis requiring arteriographic determination of the extent and severity of carotid artery disease (Figure 10.6). Arteriography is mandatory in patients who are considered candidates for carotid endarterectomy or carotid artery stenting. Additionally, patients with severe carotid artery obstructive disease and coronary artery disease requiring coronary bypass surgery have a substantially higher risk of perioperative stroke unless the carotid artery obstruction is treated before or concomitant with the coronary bypass operation. The skilled invasive cardiologist should not hesitate to study the extracranial carotid arteries in patients meeting any of the above criteria for suspected carotid artery disease.

Subclavian Arteriography

Arteriographic study of the subclavian arteries is needed to evaluate several clinical syndromes. Claudication of either of the upper extremities is generally indicative of

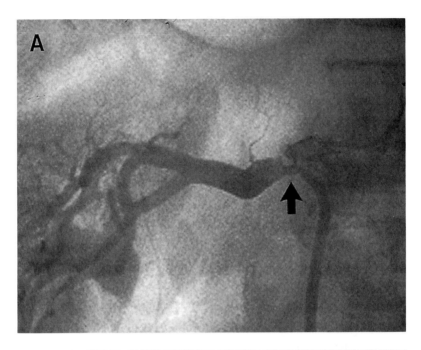

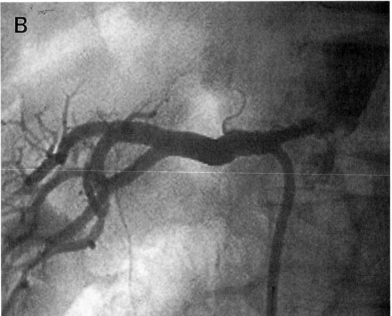

Figure 10.4. Selective right renal arteriogram in a patient presenting with accelerated hypertension. (A) A high-grade atherosclerotic stenosis at the origin of the renal artery (arrow). (B) After stent placement, the proximal renal artery appears essentially normal. This patient's hypertension was eliminated after stenting.

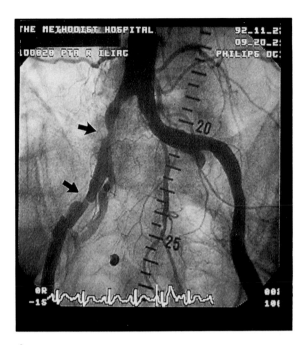

A

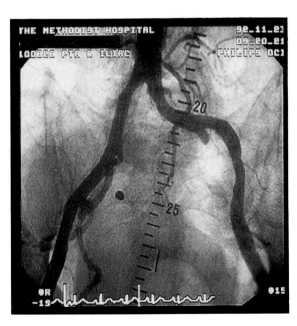

B

Figure 10.5 Abdominal aortogram showing the iliac bifurcation and both iliac arteries in a patient with right hip claudication. (A) There are severe stenoses in the right common iliac artery (upper arrow) and right external iliac artery (lower arrow). The left common and external iliac arteries are diseased but patent while the left internal iliac is occluded. (B) Following placement of two stents, the right iliac artery system is widely patent.

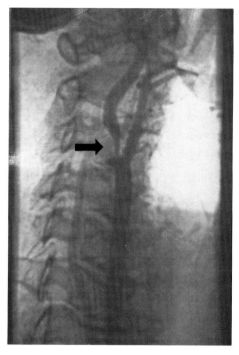

Figure 10.6. Selective carotid arteriogram in a patient being evaluated for coronary artery disease who gave a history of transient blurred vision and had a carotid bruit. There is a severe stenosis at the origin of the internal carotid artery (arrow). He subsequently underwent carotid endarterectomy at the time of coronary artery bypass surgery.

stenosis of the subclavian artery. Clinical suspicion is often enhanced by the measurement of differential blood pressure readings from the right and left arm or from a substantially lower blood pressure reading of one or both upper extremities relative to the lower extremities.

Patients who present with symptoms of vertebral basilar insufficiency may have subclavian artery stenosis as the etiology of these symptoms. Since the subclavian artery gives rise to the vertebral artery, severe stenosis at the origin or proximal segment of the subclavian artery may cause a reversal of the flow in the vertebral artery system, thus siphoning blood from the posterior circulation of the brain. This syndrome has been termed the *subclavian steal syndrome* (Figure 10.7). It behooves clinicians to recognize this entity since correction of the subclavian stenosis by interventional techniques can be readily accomplished.

For the past twenty years, coronary artery bypass surgery utilizing the internal mammary arteries has become a standard approach in the surgical treatment of coronary artery disease. Generally, the left internal mammary artery will be used to bypass the left anterior descending coronary artery. However, occasionally both the right and left internal mammary arteries will be used for left anterior descending, diagonal, or obtuse marginal artery bypass conduits. The subsequent development of myocardial ischemia in patients having received internal mammary artery bypasses may occur as a result of the development of stenosis of the proximal

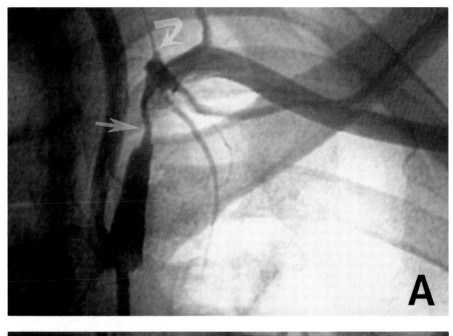

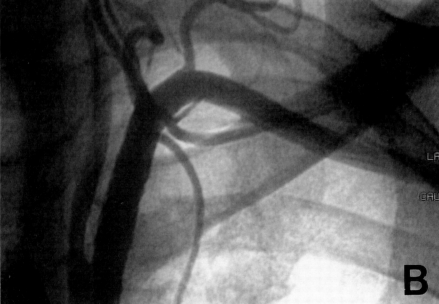

Figure 10.7. Selective left subclavian arteriogram in a patient presenting with symptoms of vertebral–basilar insufficiency. (A) There is a severe stenosis of the left subclavian artery (straight arrow) prior to any major branches. Note the absence of flow in the vertebral artery (curved arrow) and only sparse filling of the internal mammary artery (narrow arrow). (B) After PTCA and stenting of the subclavian stenosis, the vertebral and internal mammary arteries fill well. This patient's symptoms resolved.

subclavian artery.[24] The symptoms and objective manifestations of such a syndrome are indistinguishable from ischemic manifestations due to stenosis which has developed within the bypass itself or the native coronary artery. For example, a patient with a left internal mammary artery bypass to the left anterior descending may develop effort angina and manifest an ischemic response in the distribution of the left anterior descending coronary artery during thallium scintigraphy stress testing. If coronary arteriography is performed and does not show stenosis within the left internal mammary artery or the native left anterior descending coronary artery, consideration should be given to subclavian artery stenosis as the etiology of the ischemic manifestations in this patient.

CONTRAINDICATIONS

There are no absolute contraindications to peripheral angiography. As with all invasive procedures, the need to obtain the information that the procedure provides must be balanced against the likelihood for serious complications related to the procedure.

There are numerous relative contraindications, however, which must be borne in mind when evaluating a patient for angiography.[25] These include:

1. Severe prior reaction to contrast media, including hypotension and acute bronchospastic respiratory distress. If angiography is required despite such a prior history, pretreatment with corticosteroids, antihistamines, and an H_2 blocker can be administered and will generally prevent or limit the severity of the allergic reaction.

2. Impaired renal function. The potential for contrast-induced nephropathy is increased if the baseline serum creatinine is over 1.5 mg/dl and increases proportionate to the magnitude of elevation of serum creatinine. Diabetic patients with renal insufficiency are particularly prone to develop contrast nephropathy. Preventive measures to limit renal damage include maximizing hydration prior to dye delivery and the use of calcium channel blocking agents.

3. Coagulapathy due to hematologic disorders or secondary to drug administration (e.g., warfarin). A prothrombin time of more than 3 or 4 sec above control values invites the potential for bleeding at the arterial access site. In general, angiography can be safely performed in the presence of antiplatelet agents such as aspirin and ticlopidine, although more intensive hemostasis maneuvers may be required when the catheter and sheaths are removed, such as prolonged arterial pressure.

4. Hemodynamic or cardiac instability such as hypotension and serious arrhythmias. Efforts should be made to stabilize the patient's hemodynamics and optimally control arrhythmias before angiography is carried out.

5. Major electrolyte imbalance, such as severe hypokalemia. Improvement or correction of the electrolyte abnormality should be undertaken before the angiography is done.

6. Inability to lie flat on the angiography table due to respiratory insufficiency or congestive heart failure. Propping the patient's head up and treatment of the underlying respiratory distress will usually allow angiographic studies to be ultimately undertaken.

COMPLICATIONS

In qualified hands, the safety of noncardiac angiography is well established. Nevertheless, the potential for both minor and serious complications exists.[25,26]

The most common complications are those related to the puncture site.[27] These include hemorrhage requiring transfusion, thrombosis, pseudoaneurysm formation, arteriovenous fistula, and loss of limb. The likelihood of one of these complications occurring is approximately 0.5%.

Systemic reactions including pulmonary edema and cardiac arrest, hypotension, transient ischemic events, or stroke are rare but major potential consequences of angiography. The incidence of death is very low (0.03% to 0.05%) and is most likely to occur in patients with fragile hemodynamics such as in those with acute aortic dissections.[25]

Catheter and guidewire-related complications may occur. These include perforation with dye extravasation outside the confines of the artery, distal embolization, and catheter or guidewire breakage.

Idiosyncratic contrast reactions may vary from mild, such as a rash, to anaphylactic reactions. Death due to contrast reactions is extremely rare and is estimated to occur in fewer than one per 20,000 patients. Contrast nephropathy is of concern in any patient with renal dysfunction,[3,4,28] particularly diabetes. Pretreatment with fluid hydration and calcium channel blockers and the use of nonionic contrast media reduces the incidence and severity of this complication.

ADVANTAGES AND DISADVANTAGES

Various imaging modalities may provide valuable information which overlaps with that which could be acquired by angiography.

A diagnosis of aortic aneurysm and aortic dissection can be made by computed tomography, magnetic resonance imaging, and ultrasound imaging. Each of these may provide diagnostic information and obviate the need for angiography. However, angiography is invaluable in assessing blood flow, particularly to branch vessels. Such information is crucial to plan the correct operation.

The diagnosis of renal artery stenosis may be suggested by nuclear imaging methods and ultrasound imaging of the renal arteries. However, none of these tests can supplant angiography for definitive evaluation of the location and severity of renal artery stenosis.

Ultrasound of the carotid arteries at the bifurcation of the common carotid arteries is a valuable screening tool. However, angiography is necessary in almost all patients in whom carotid artery surgery is being contemplated. Refinements in magnetic resonance angiography have markedly enhanced the capability of this noninvasive imaging modality to access the severity of extracranial cerebral vascular stenoses.

Evaluation of peripheral vascular disease involving the lower extremities requires angiographic assessment. While other techniques are available to assess general flow impairment to the lower limbs, angiography can precisely pinpoint the location and severity of disease better than any less invasive technique. This is particularly true of the more peripheral vessels such as those below the knee.

FUTURE ADVANCEMENT

Dramatic refinements in x-ray technology and angiographic techniques have greatly improved the safety and utility of noncardiac angiography over the past decade. Digital imaging methodologies have increased the diagnostic capabilities of angiographic techniques while improving the safety of these procedures by allowing the use of smaller catheters and less contrast media. Further refinements are very likely in the future.

Despite the sophistication of angiographic methods and the potential for further future improvement, the use of less invasive imaging methods as a substitute for angiography is gaining momentum as a substitute for the more invasive angiographic techniques. It is likely that these more noninvasive approaches will supersede angiography as the definitive diagnostic test in many of the disease entities cited in this chapter. Until then, angiography remains the mainstay of diagnosis of central and peripheral vascular disease states.

REFERENCES

1. Forssmann W: Die Sondierung des rechten Herzens. *Klin Wochnschr* 8:2085, 1929.
2. Seldinger SI: Catheter replacement of the needle in percutaneous arteriography: a new technique. *Acta Radiol* (Stockh) 39:368, 1953.
3. ACC Cardiovascular Imaging Committee: Use of nonionic or low-osmolar contrast agents in cardiovascular procedures. *J Am Coll Cardiol* 21:269–273, 1993.
4. Bettmann MA, Higgins CB: Comparison of an ionic with a nonionic contrast agent for cardiac angiography. *Cardiac Angiog* 29:S70–S74, 1985.
5. Gishen P, Lakier JB: The ascending aorta in aortic stenosis. *Cardiovasc Radiol* 2:85, 1979.
6. Williams JCP, Barratt-Boyes BG, Lowe JB: Supravalvular aortic stenosis. *Circulation* 24:1311, 1961.
7. Taubman JO, Goodman DJ, Steiner RE: The value of contrast studies in the investigation of aortic valve disease. *Clin Radiol* 17:23, 1966.
8. Cohn LH, Mason DT, Ross J, et al: Preoperative assessment of aortic regurgitation in patients with mitral valve disease. *Am J Cardiol* 19:177–182, 1967.
9. Sprayregen S: Radiologic spectrum of arteriosclerotic aneurysms of aortic arch. *NY State J Med* 78:2198, 1978.
10. Hirst AE Jr, Gore I: Marfan's syndrome: a review. *Prog Cardiovasc Dis* 16:187, 1973.
11. DeBakey ME, Henly WS, Cooley DA, et al: Surgical management of dissecting aneurysms of the aorta. *J Thorac Cardiovasc Surg* 49:130, 1965.
12. Dinsmore RE, Willerson JT, Buckley MJ: Dissecting aneurysm of the aorta. Aortographic features affecting prognosis. *Diagn Radiol* 105:567, 1972.

13. Shuford WH, Sybers RG, Weens HS: Problems of the aortographic diagnosis of dissecting aneurysms of the aorta. *N Engl J Med* 280:225, 1969.

14. Kimbris D, Iskandrian AS, Segal EL, et al: Anomalous aortic origin of coronary arteries. *Circulation* 58:606, 1978.

15. Welton DE, Young JB, Raizner AE, et al: The value and safety of cardiac catheterization during active infective endocarditis. *Am J Cardiol* 44:1306, 1979.

16. Weisman AD, Adams RD: Neurological complications of dissecting aortic aneurysm. *Brain* 67:69, 1944.

17. Shinebourne EA, Tam ASY, Elsee AM, et al: Coarctation of the aorta in infancy and childhood. *Br Heart J* 38:375, 1976.

18. Fleming AW, Green DC: Traumatic aneurysms of the thoracic aorta: report of 43 patients. *Ann Thorac Surg* 18:91, 1974.

19. Marsh DG, Sturm JT: Traumatic aortic rupture: roentgenographic indications for angiography. *Ann Thorac Surg* 21:337, 1976.

20. Brewster DC, Retana A, Waltman AC, et al: Angiography in the management of aneurysms of the abdominal aorta: its value and safety. *N Engl J Med* 292:822, 1975.

21. Eyler WR, Clark MD, Garmon JE, et al: Angiography of the renal areas including a comparative study of renal arterial stenoses in patients with and without hypertension. *Radiology* 78:879, 1962.

22. Bookstein JJ, Abrams HL, Buenger RE, et al: Radiologic aspects of renovascular hypertension. Part 3. Appraisal of arteriography. *JAMA* 21:368, 1972.

23. vanBreda A, Katzen BT: Cerebrovascular disease. In: vanBreda A, Katzen BT (eds): Digital subtraction angiography: practical aspects. Thorofare, NJ: Slack Inc, 1986.

24. McIvor ME, Williams GM, Brinker J: Subclavian coronary steal through a LIMA-to-LAD bypass graft. *Cathet Cardiovasc Diagn* 14:100–104, 1988.

25. Kandarpa K, Gardiner GA Jr: Angiography. In Kandarpa K, Aruny JE: *Handbook of Interventional Radiologic Procedures*, Boston, Little, Brown, 1996, pp 3–26.

26. Hessel SJ, Adams DF, Abrams HL: Complications of angiography. *Radiology* 138:273–281, 1981.

27. Barnes RW, Petersen JL, Krugmire RB, et al: Complications of percutaneous femoral arterial catheterization: prospective evaluation with the Doppler ultrasonic velocity detector. *Am J Cardiol* 33:259–263, 1974.

28. Lautin EM, Freeman NJ, Shoenfeld AH, et al: Radiocontrast-associated renal dysfunction: incidence and risk factors. *AJR* 157:49–58, 1991.

Index

ISBN 0-89640-318-1